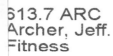

teach®
yourself

fitness
jeff archer

For over 60 years, more than
40 million people have learnt over
750 subjects the **teach yourself**
way, with impressive results.

be where you want to be
with **teach yourself**

Thanks to Independent Newspapers for permission to use source material for the exercise section of this book.

Illustrations by Barking Dog Art.

For UK order enquiries: please contact Bookpoint Ltd, 130 Milton Park, Abingdon, Oxon OX14 4SB. Telephone: +44 (0) 1235 827720. Fax: +44 (0) 1235 400454. Lines are open 09.00–18.00, Monday to Saturday, with a 24-hour message answering service. Details about our titles and how to order are available at www.teachyourself.co.uk

For USA order enquiries: please contact McGraw-Hill Customer Services, PO Box 545, Blacklick, OH 43004-0545, USA. Telephone: 1-800-722-4726. Fax: 1-614-755-5645.

For Canada order enquiries: please contact McGraw-Hill Ryerson Ltd, 300 Water St, Whitby, Ontario L1N 9B6, Canada. Telephone: 905 430 5000. Fax: 905 430 5020.

Long renowned as the authoritative source for self-guided learning – with more than 40 million copies sold worldwide – the **teach yourself** series includes over 300 titles in the fields of languages, crafts, hobbies, business, computing and education.

British Library Cataloguing in Publication Data: a catalogue record for this title is available from the British Library.

Library of Congress Catalog Card Number: on file.

First published in UK 2006 by Hodder Education, 338 Euston Road, London, NW1 3BH.

First published in US 2006 by Contemporary Books, a Division of the McGraw-Hill Companies, 1 Prudential Plaza, 130 East Randolph Street, Chicago, IL 60601 USA.

This edition published 2006.

The **teach yourself** name is a registered trade mark of Hodder Headline.

Typeset by Transet Limited, Coventry, England.
Printed in Great Britain for Hodder Education, a division of Hodder Headline, 338 Euston Road, London NW1 3BH, by Cox & Wyman Ltd, Reading, Berkshire.

Hodder Headline's policy is to use papers that are natural, renewable and recyclable products and made from wood grown in sustainable forests. The logging and manufacturing processes are expected to conform to the environmental regulations of the country of origin.

Impression number   10 9 8 7 6 5 4 3 2 1
Year   2010 2009 2008 2007 2006

contents

dedication

Teach Yourself Fitness is dedicated to everyone who wants to feel fitter, healthier, happier and enjoy living to the full. If life is fun now, imagine how much better it will be with the body you want, the fitness you've always dreamed of and energy you never thought you'd have.

Deciding to read *Teach Yourself Fitness* is the right choice. This book will help you experiment with some exciting new approaches and enjoy your journey and the results it brings.

Results like these, from people who have followed our approach already:

I feel fitter than I have done in years.

I have more energy, I exercise more and I have lost a stone in weight.

My diet is 100 times better.

I'm much more motivated to exercise now.

I've experienced renewed energy.

I now eat at regular intervals, drink more water, eat more fruit and drink less alcohol.

Keeping fit and healthy is an issue that affects everyone. As long as you have your health, you can cope with anything. But how do you go about reaching and maintaining the level of fitness that suits you? How do you ensure that you are always performing to the best of your abilities?

Teach Yourself Fitness shows you how to design your own unique fitness routine and food plan that will get you the results you want throughout your life.

The benefits of improved fitness are simple. If you take regular exercise and eat sensibly you can:

• Manage your weight effectively
• Determine your body shape
• Regulate your blood pressure
• Reduce your cholesterol level
• Reduce your risk of cancer
• Strengthen your heart
• Improve your mental health.

In addition to these medical benefits, those who exercise regularly and pay attention to what they eat report having a strong sense of general well-being, great energy for their daily routine, regular and quality sleep patterns, and an optimistic outlook on life. Knowing all of this, surely we must all be taking positive steps to fit fitness into our lives, mustn't we?

Apparently not. Information on fitness is everywhere and each week there seem to be new and wonderful solutions to getting fit more quickly with increasingly innovative forms of exercise and activity. For the majority of the population, fitness is often on their minds, they read about it a lot and talk about it even more, but when it comes to taking practical steps to improving fitness, things are not quite so easy.

The fitness industry started in the studio with aerobics, and in the gym with good old-fashioned pumping iron. Before this, of course, there was not much need for a fitness 'industry' as everyone kept fit through moving around as part of their daily routine. Then our lives became more sedentary and we had to think about ways in which we could add back some of the activity.

We had step classes, boxing classes, martial arts classes, spinning, circuits and indoor rowing classes to get the body going. People then looked to balance their exertions by incorporating some older, more relaxing and contemplative activities such as Yoga, Pilates, Tai Chi and massage. Within all the different disciplines, everyone has an opinion on what works best, what is most effective and what is most fun. Now there are so many options, many people do not know where to begin.

A similar story is true for diets. The benefits of eating well are clear, yet it seems that we still have not quite worked out how best to plan our food intake to suit our modern lives. Almost every day there are new suggestions of how we can eat differently for increased energy, a better body, better skin and a longer and happier life. Surely eating sensibly can't be this complicated, can it?

> With all the information out there on keeping fit and eating well, shouldn't it be easy for everyone to follow at least some of this advice and achieve the fitness they want?

We still spend far more time talking about and worrying about exercising and eating healthily than we do actually taking exercise, choosing the food we know we should choose, and avoiding the things we know are harmful to us.

One difficulty appears to be that we simply have too much information to choose from. Because there are so many different approaches, we tend to choose one, usually the newest one, the one claiming the fastest results or requiring the smallest effort, give it a go for a while, realize it does not quite fit our lives, and then move on to the next. The problem with trying all these different plans is that we never seem to settle into a routine and get the results we want. And if we do not see the results we want, we tend to give up.

Teach Yourself Fitness will help you put an end to this way of living.

Make your own plans

It is true to say that every exercise and food plan works for someone, somewhere. But these 'off-the-shelf' solutions, cannot work for everyone, all of the time. So, rather than trying each one in turn in an attempt to find the one that works best for you, why not create your own unique solution?

'It will take too long' is the usual objection, but finding out what works for you is a lot quicker than you may think. And planning your own route to success is certainly quicker than ploughing through all of the hundreds of thousands of exercise and diet books currently on the market.

If you take the time to discover what works for you, you will know that you have routines that get you results. No more wondering whether fancy tactics will help you reach your goals or not, you will have your winning strategies in place and ready to be put into action. No more shooting in the dark with what works and what doesn't. You will know what you need to do at specific times in your life, and you will know that your programmes are fun and rewarding because you will have created them that way.

Most people want to know the quickest and most painless way to get fit.

> The simple truth is that the quickest route to fitness is the one you enjoy the most.

If you enjoy fitness, you will make it part of your everyday life and you will get great results without ever feeling like you have had to make too much of an effort or put yourself out. If you get results, you will see the benefits of what you are doing and you will be keen to do more of it.

Teach Yourself Fitness is about making exercise and food fun again. Enjoying fitness so that you always guarantee maximum results, for now and for the future, with minimum frustration along the way. This book will show you how to enhance your everyday life through the benefits of regular exercise and healthy eating, without compromising on the things you like to do.

Sounds good doesn't it?

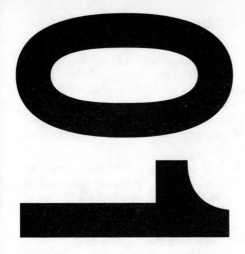

01

the world of exercise: how to make it work for you

In this chapter you will learn:
- to look at fitness in a new way
- the importance of planning, doing and reviewing
- key questions to ask when starting out.

What is different about this book?

Most fitness books focus on the facts of exercise and healthy eating. For exercise you will usually find an outline of cardiovascular fitness, strength training and flexibility. Some will venture into more recent areas of development within the fitness industry such as core training for good posture and to protect your back, stability and balance exercises for fluid movement, and functional training for particular sports and activities.

The majority of diet books will cover carbohydrates, proteins, fat, fruit and vegetables, fluid intake, the balance between all of these dietary components, and the timing of drinks and meals. In most cases, the balance between the different food groups and the timing of meals will depend on the preference of the author or the latest research on which the book is based.

Teach Yourself Fitness takes a slightly different approach. You need to know about all of the above areas of fitness and we will give you the facts so that you can operate with full knowledge of how to proceed safely. Then we take a step back from the traditional approaches to fitness and food in an effort to show you how you can get better results, faster. We will show you how to simplify your whole approach by ensuring your success before you take your first deep exercise breath or bite of healthy eating.

This book begins with the assumption that, given a little prompting, everyone knows roughly what they should and should not do with regard to taking exercise and putting food into their mouths. We have been exposed to so many magazine articles and television programmes, that it is not a case of having enough information, the tricky thing is to know what to do with it. In our modern world, the information we receive each day on exercise and diets can reach overload point so the last thing you need is more information along the same lines.

What you really need are new techniques to help you incorporate all of this information into your life. This book forms a guide to how you can take all the knowledge available and make it work for you. It is a blueprint for designing your own tailor-made fitness and food plan and putting your plans into action. *A guide that acts as your very own expert Personal Trainer.*

What do I do first?

To help you reach your own personal success with fitness and nutrition, we will look at the three really important elements of exercise and diet – planning, doing and reviewing.

Step 1 Plan

Sounds obvious and sounds boring, doesn't it? Why would you want to plan when you can just get on with it? Well, think about your previous attempts at exercising and dieting. Did you plan? Did you succeed? If you did plan, how much planning did you do? How long did your success last for? Has more detailed planning ever led you to better success in the past?

> We are talking about proper, thorough planning here. Planning to the end point. Not just planning to get fit, but planning the details of *how* you get fit.

I know, the thought of it is already putting you off, but really, do you think you will get the true success you deserve without proper consideration of how it is all going to pan out? If you think hard enough you will probably be able to anticipate the points in the future where your good intentions could get tripped up, and the thought of planning around these turns you off the whole idea of getting fit. Do not push these thoughts away. If you are anticipating these problems and you do not give them due consideration now, they *will* trip you up. If you can overcome them immediately in your head with some creative planning, you will sail through them when they crop up for real.

Rarely are great things achieved without due consideration at the beginning of the project. Architects do not just plan to build an office block, they draw up detailed drawings of each progressive point of the process, from idea to completed structure on the paper. They know what has to happen at every stage, who will be involved and when they will be needed, and what the possible pitfalls could be. All this before a brick is laid. When we cook new dishes for the first time, we follow recipes – where would we be without them? Sure, you may adapt dishes to suit your taste once you have made them a few times, but for the first time out, you need as much guidance as you can get. You need precise instructions on what to do at each stage of the process, what to look for and what to avoid.

So when we talk about planning, we mean detailed, thorough, carefully considered plans that take us from the beginning to the end of what we want to achieve. You will have examples from your own life when planning something well led to great success. The success of your new regime depends on the same key elements, so give planning due consideration and the progress to follow will be smooth and swift.

Step 2 Do

Sounds even more obvious, doesn't it? But you will know from personal experience that taking exercise and eating healthily are often easier said than done. And when pushed, we can come up with all sorts of excuses as to why we should not go to the gym today. Suddenly that report you have been procrastinating over all day becomes of vital importance and you cannot think about anything else until you have done it. Or you really must meet up with your best friend. She has been having a tough time recently and could do with seeing you for a good chat to cheer her up. We are also very creative with our reasons for making choices on what we eat and drink. We can easily talk ourselves into glossing over various food vices if we deserve a little 'treat'. And how many times have you overheard someone who 'deserved that extra glass of wine as it really had been a very tough day'?

> Having taken the time to work out your plan that will lead you to the fitness and the figure you want, give it a chance. Do it, and do it now, not later.

Follow the plan that you have taken the trouble to create. Do what you know will work for you and be diligent in avoiding what you know will hamper your progress. This is not a project in creative excuse making or affirming that there are too many distractions in life for you to achieve the body you want. Those projects are easy and you have probably been quite successful at them up until now.

What is required from here on is the fortitude to take the action you know is required to get the results you want. Only you can do it so do not delay any longer.

Step 3 Review

This is your chance to stand out from the crowd. If you plan and do, you will achieve results. Whether or not those results are enough for you, is up to you. If they are, great, you can continue in the same vein. If not, you have the opportunity to modify your approach to create greater success.

Faced with results that are different from what they expected, or not quite what they hoped for, many people fall into the trap of taking the view that the whole plan is not working. They have 'failed' again so they go back to what they were doing before. But why is this pattern of behaviour so common? The old routine did not give you the results you wanted before, so why would you want to go back to it now?

Going 'back to the drawing board' feels like a negative experience and gives you the sense that, though you tried something different, it was not good enough. Or, worse than that, *you* were not good enough. Often you can console yourself that you will start again on Monday but there is a danger that each successive new start on Monday will be more difficult than the last until one new week arrives when you cannot be bothered to even try any more.

An easier and more effective way to deal with the situation is not to give up on your new regime completely, but instead to analyse what has worked best and do more of it. Pick out the good bits and expand them. Isolate what does not suit you so well and change that bit only, not the whole thing. With regular review, you gradually develop a finely tuned approach that really works for you. While others are struggling with their old patterns of behaviour and trying different approaches every week, you will be forging ahead with a new, improved and regularly reviewed plan for personal success.

What is the most important thing to do?

To begin with, allocate one-third of your time and effort to each of the key stages of planning, doing and reviewing. All three are crucial and with an even balance between the three you will achieve your aims quickly and easily. Yes this approach requires a little more thought and consideration than you may have wanted to give to your fitness when you set out, but consider what is important here – results. If you want results and you want them quickly, you know that a little bit of time and some brain power are small investments for what will be exciting rewards.

Over time you will become more and more familiar with what you need to do, and when you need to do it in order to achieve specific results. You will need less time for planning and reviewing and you can use this extra time for doing. And the more time you spend on doing effective activities, the better your results will be.

So, how do you go about finding an exercise routine that suits you, your needs and your lifestyle? How can you fast-track yourself to the results that you want and deserve, without feeling that you have had to turn your life upside down?

Do not over-complicate fitness

First you must establish what you want to achieve with your fitness programme. To make it easy and avoid being overwhelmed, begin with just one key aim that you feel you must make happen. It has to be something you really want, something that you would feel disappointed if you never managed to achieve as long as you lived.

Explore why you want success in this area. Hoping to achieve something because it would be 'nice' to have it, or because you feel you should do it, or even because someone else thought it would be a good idea if you did it, simply makes your life difficult. Your goals must have clear reasoning behind them and it must be your reasoning to stand any chance of success.

Decide on a realistic time by which you will have reached this goal. Not an abstract idea of when something might happen, but a carefully considered plan that takes into account everything and everyone else that you have in your life, and incorporates your fitness goal as a priority within this structure.

Highlight what you will do to make your goal a reality. What exercises and activities will become part of your life? When will these activities take place? What changes will you make to your diet? Are there any other alterations that you will need to make to your lifestyle? Who might be affected by the changes you are proposing and how will you deal with these situations?

Finally, pick your starting point. Isolate the first practical steps on the road to the new you and choose when you will take them. Choose specific days and times for putting these steps into action and stick to them. And remember, there is no time like the present. What can you do right now to set you on your way to achieving your goals?

Here is a real-life example of this process.

Name: Deborah

Date: 2 December, 2004

One Key Fitness Aim
To be able to fit into my favourite size 12 jeans.

Why do I want to achieve this goal?
It has been four years since I wore these jeans comfortably. I try them on regularly hoping that they will fit but knowing deep down that they won't. I cannot believe it has been so long since I was the right size for these jeans and I would hate to think I will never get into them again. I really want to fit into them as they give me loads of options in my wardrobe. They also represent a positive period of my life. I wore them on some great nights out and life at that time was really fun. I bought them when I knew I was in the best shape of my life and I really enjoyed feeling that way each day. If I can get back into these jeans, I know I will feel happier and more confident.

By what date will you have achieved this goal?
I would like to be into the jeans for the beginning of the New Year but I know that will be difficult with the usual routine of work, social and family commitments at Christmas time. With all that in mind, if I knew I was on the way to reaching my goal and could get there by the end of February, I would be happy. We are going away for half term at the end of February and I would love to be able to take the jeans with me and wear them on holiday.

What will you do to ensure you reach your goal?
To begin with I will need to exercise three or four times each week and I think a combination of using the gym and the swimming pool would suit me best. I also need to fit more activity into my daily routine by taking a walk either before work or at lunchtimes. I will eat a little less at mealtimes, think about the snacks that I eat and reduce the amount of alcohol I drink each week. I can eat more healthily at mealtimes if I cook something slightly different for myself than the food the kids are eating. Actually, I think I will make all our meals slightly healthier which will be good for the children and my husband. I will need to be careful about how much I change everything or I could have a rebellion on my hands.

When will you start with the New You?

Today is Thursday so I can start this lunchtime by taking a walk to the supermarket where I can buy something fresh for this evening's meal. I will think about some healthier food options tomorrow night in preparation for shopping on Saturday. On Sunday we can go to the health club. If I go a bit earlier than everyone else I can make a start in the gym, my husband can bring the children for a swim and I will join them later in the pool. Next week I will go to the gym on Monday lunchtime and Wednesday after work and aim to get back there at the weekend. Right now I will get a bottle of water to see me through the day, throw out the crisps in my desk drawer and replace them with some fruit or some plain nuts.

Already you can see how, by taking the time to plan, some new ideas and opportunities for acting on your intentions present themselves for consideration. Now run through the questions for yourself. Consider what new options for achieving your goals you have by the end of the process that you did not have when you started.

Getting started

Name:

....

Date:

....

Key Fitness Aim

....

....

Why do I want to achieve this goal?

....

....

By what date will I have achieved this goal?

....

....

When will I start with the New Me?

....

....

What will I do to ensure I reach my goal?

....

....

....

....

Sounds simple doesn't it? Answer a few easy questions and off you go towards everything you ever wanted from your fitness. So why is it that not everyone can achieve their fitness aims when they want to?

There are a number of common reasons why people become frustrated with exercise and food:

- They lack the correct motivation to begin.
- They expect complete results immediately.
- They lose motivation along the way.
- They choose an impossible plan.
- They fall foul of injury or illness.

You can ensure that you do not suffer from any of these frustrations by examining each of them in turn and dealing with them right now.

02

overcoming obstacles to get the results you want

In this chapter you will learn:
- to recognize common fitness pitfalls
- how to make sure they do not happen to you
- positive strategies for guaranteed results.

Finding your true motivation

Fitness Pitfall 1: Lacking the correct motivation to begin

Usual Outcome: Giving up on dreams before getting properly started

The Road to Success: Finding your true motivation

So why do you want things to be different? What is your motivation for embarking on your new fitness regime? It had better be good because it has got to sustain you during the coming months and keep you on track. Do you know where to get motivation from and how to find it when you need it most?

Motivation isn't something you can hold in your hands, it is not tangible. It is not even the same for everyone. But one thing you can be sure of, you are going to need it if you are to make the changes necessary to reach your fitness goals. So how do we get motivated?

To give yourself the best chance of success, you must decide what you really, really want. True motivation doesn't come from deciding what you could do, or what you should do, or what someone else thinks would be good for you, but from what you really want to do.

Think about it now. What are the three things you really want to achieve with your fitness? What are the things you would really regret if you did not make them happen? If you were to broadcast to the world in six months' time, what would you want to tell them you had achieved with your fitness between now and then?

Now write them down:

My Fitness Goals

Priority 1:

Priority 2:

Priority 3:

Now let's look a little more closely at the priorities to ensure they are the right goals to be striving for, and to give you the best possible chance of success.

Take control of your own fitness future

You may be familiar with the concept of SMART goals. SMART is an acronym used in the fitness world and beyond to consolidate aims and objectives. For an increased chance of success, your goals should be:

- Specific
- Measurable
- Achievable
- Realistic
- Time-framed.

We can illustrate setting SMART goals with the following example.

Name: James

Date: February 2005

My Fitness Goals
Priority 1: To take more exercise

Priority 2: To take part in a running event

Priority 3: To decrease my waist measurement by one inch

Let's look at how we can turn one of James's fitness priorities into a SMART goal by examining Priority 2 in more detail.

What is my fitness priority?
To take part in a running event.

Be Specific
Write out all details of your fitness priority to make your goal as specific as possible.

When would you like to take part in an event?
Before the end of this year.

What type of event would you like to take part in?
A 10 km road race.

Where would you like the event to be?
In a countryside area, not too far from home.

What kind of route would you like to run?
A quiet scenic route, without too many hills.

How long do you want the run to take?
Around 60 minutes.

Is it Measurable?
Describe how you will measure your success with your fitness priority.

I will be able to run greater distances and for a longer time. I will feel more comfortable with these increased times and distances over the coming weeks and months. I will know I am succeeding when I can enter an event with confidence, and look forward to it as it approaches. Then I will take part in the event, enjoy it and complete it.

Is it Achievable?
Is your fitness priority truly achievable by you?

I used to run a lot and enjoy it. I have had some problems with my knees over the years but am confident that if I train carefully, increase my running gradually and do not overdo it, I will be able to achieve this goal.

Is it Realistic?
Is your chosen fitness priority realistic given your current life circumstances?

Work is busy and I do have to travel quite a lot, but running is portable and if I look at my schedule carefully each week I will be able to plan times to exercise.

Make it Time-framed
Select a time by which your fitness priority will, without any doubt, be reached.

In my mind, I would like to run an event while the weather is still good – I am not a big fan of the colder weather. With this in mind, I am committed to completing my 10 km run by the end of October this year.

Clearly, setting SMART goals helps explore your objectives and how they will be realized in more detail. The questions that you will ask yourself surrounding your own fitness objectives will bring you to a greater understanding of what needs to be done and the action you need to take to guarantee progress. This in turn increases your chances of success.

Take a minute now to make one of your fitness priorities a SMART goal.

What is my fitness priority?

....

Be Specific

Write out all details of your fitness priority to make your goal as specific as possible.

....

....

Is it Measurable?

Describe how you will measure your success with your fitness priority.

....

....

Is it Achievable?

Is your fitness priority truly achievable by you?

....

....

Is it Realistic?

Is your chosen fitness priority realistic given your current life circumstances?

....

....

Make it Time-framed

Select a time by which your fitness priority will, without any doubt, be reached.

....

....

So now you have a much clearer idea of where you are heading with your fitness. But how can you absolutely guarantee that you reach your objectives and achieve exactly what you are aiming for?

The following process takes slightly longer than setting SMART goals but it is well worth the investment of time as your results will be dramatic. As with many things in life, the devil is in the detail and the more detail you can create around what it is you want to achieve and why, the more likely you will be to succeed.

Firstly, **state your goal as a positive** and make it something exciting to aim for. Knowing that you want to lose weight is fine, but understanding what your target weight will be and what this will mean for your life, what opportunities this will offer you, what outfits this will allow you to wear and how you will feel when you have achieved the result, is even more motivating.

Next you must establish **where you are now** in relation to your goal. You must clearly understand the gap between your current situation and your desired situation, in order that you can set a truly realistic time frame for the achievement.

Now ask yourself, **'what will I see, hear and feel when I reach my goal?'** Giving yourself the opportunity to flesh out a picture of what reaching this goal will enable you to do, feel, see and hear allows you to imagine living as if you have already succeeded. Your brain begins working on new and positive thought patterns, you can sense success in your head and in you body. These positive thought patterns are a great asset in the quest to begin making the dream come true.

Then ask yourself, **'how will I know when I have achieved my goal?'** This is a crucial question to ask so that you are completely clear on when you will reach your current objectives. This allows you to feel the sense of achievement and success that you deserve. It is fine to reset some new goals at this point, but ensure that you enjoy the moment of victory before moving on. If you do not establish how you will know when you have achieved your goal well in advance, the tendency is to keep moving the goalposts. This may lead to you feeling like you never succeed, despite the fact that you may have hit your initial targets and gone beyond them ages ago.

The next question to ask yourself is, **'what will reaching this goal get for me?'** It is important that you recognize what achieving a goal will get for you, and also what it won't get for you, at an early stage, to avoid disappointment later. People sometimes make giant mental leaps to associate losing weight with being completely happy, enjoying life at all times and sometimes even finding a new partner. If all this does not happen they may become frustrated. Make sure that you know that hitting your target fitness level or weight may get you many things, but not necessarily a new lover! Focus on what it will definitely get you, not what it might lead to.

Then confirm that the goal is **an idea created by you and for you.** Self-generated goals are almost always achieved more effectively than a goal that someone else has suggested. Individuals can shed half their body weight if they decide that they need to make some drastic changes. Others may fail to shift a pound if it is someone else who has 'suggested' they need to slim down a bit and not their own choice to do so.

Find out what **resources you will need** to reach your goal. Whether it be a gym membership, a pair of trainers, some time to yourself, family support, some dumbbells, or even time to read a book like this one, you must be clear on precisely what you need to put in place to ensure success, and when you will need these resources. The last thing you want is to be tripped up half way to your goal by something simple that you could have anticipated well ahead of time.

Along the same lines, you must establish if there is **any cost to anyone else** of you achieving your goal. If a by-product of you embarking on a fitness programme is that you spend more time out of the house away from your partner, you must consider how this will affect them. If you choose your specific weight loss programme, there might be a completely different kind of food in stock in the house which may have implications for your family. You need to be fully aware of these issues and able to anticipate a way around them before causing chaos at home.

Finally ask, **is your goal truly exciting, compelling and desirable** to you? If it is not then perhaps you need to add more detail to some of the questions above. Only when the goal appears really exciting and totally enthralling can you guarantee success.

By creating SMART goals you can drastically increase your chances of success. Then, by checking your ideas with the more detailed questions, you will have fully explored your aims and objectives and how they fit into your life.

This allows you to feel true motivation to succeed. You now have the best possible chance of making your fitness dreams and desires a reality. Try it now and see how exciting you can make your goals.

Making your fitness dreams a reality

State your aims in the positive.

....

....

Where am I now?

....

....

What will I see, hear and feel when I reach my goal?

....

....

How will I know when I have achieved my goal?

....

....

What will reaching this goal get for me?

....

....

Is this goal created by me, for me?

....

....

What resources will I need to reach my goal?

....

....

Is there a cost to anyone else of me achieving my goal?

....

....

Is my goal truly exciting, compelling and desirable to me?

....

....

Patience is a virtue

Fitness Pitfall 2: Expecting complete results immediately

Usual Outcome: Slower than expected progress leading to loss of motivation

The Road to Success: Patience is a virtue

Wanting and expecting instant results from a new fitness routine or nutrition plan is one of the main reasons why people do not reach their intended goals and soon give up trying. They expect too much too soon, and when they do not get it they think things are not working and revert back to their old familiar habits. It is important to consider at this stage, the planning stage, how we can avoid falling into a trap where all your good intentions fizzle out to nothing.

It is crucial to be honest with yourself, your current situation, what you can realistically expect to achieve and by when.

No one ever put on a stone of body fat overnight, but often people expect to lose this much weight in an instant. Is this being realistic? Consider how long it may have taken for the extra pounds to have crept on. Think candidly about when you last lived a lifestyle that was completely at one with staying in shape and feeling fit. It may have been a while ago.

When we were young, we ran around all day without ever feeling tired but gradually our levels of daily activity have decreased. Our modern day lifestyles have led us to walk around 25 miles less each week than we did 20 years ago, and labour-saving devices mean that we do not burn nearly as many calories as we used to in our daily routine. Is it right then to expect to achieve a lean-bodied, high-energy lifestyle within a matter of days?

Whatever you set out to achieve with your fitness, you have to think about when you can realistically expect to see results. If you are too impatient, you will be disappointed. If you are honest with yourself about what you can achieve and by when, you will be pleasantly surprised at each stage of your progress.

Even before you start doing anything physical, a helpful mental exercise is to sit down and spend a few moments imagining how your new fitness regime is going to unfold. Your goal may be to run a marathon, hit your target weight or simply to exercise regularly. Whatever it is, take some time to think how things are going to work out before you start. Take a moment right now to begin visualizing your route to success.

Top tip – Exercise your brain before you exercise your body.

- Find a quiet place where you will not be disturbed.
- Think about what you are about to achieve.
- Consider your goal in relation to where you are now.
- Focus on the differences between the way you live now and the way you will be living when you have reached your goal and are maintaining a new lifestyle.
- Think about how long it will take you to make all of the changes involved in moving from one lifestyle to the other.

- Now make an informed decision on a date by which you will have achieved your goal.
- Finally, allow yourself a reasonable 'grace period' by adding an extra week or two to your schedule in order to allow for all unforeseen circumstances.
- The date you arrive at now is the date by which you will be living a different life.

If we stop to think about our goals properly, most of us will know approximately how long we will need to reach them, given our current situation and lifestyle. The reason many people set unrealistic dates for achieving goals is that they imagine they do not want to wait for success. They want it now, they want it instantly, and nothing else will do.

Unfortunately, the most common result of impatience with a fitness plan is that by not allowing sufficient time to develop new habits and by not giving our bodies time to adjust and show us some progress, we become frustrated. If we do not see the results we want immediately, we lose sight of why we started the programme in the first place and we give up. If we feel motivated, we might begin the same plan again the following week. Or we may choose a different plan to work on for a new week. This pattern of repeated sweeping changes can lead to our bodies being confused by different routines. Ironically, this can ultimately end up with us achieving the opposite of the situation we were aiming for. In the absence of a measured approach, our 'stop – start' good intentions can leave us fatter and less fit than ever before.

You have heard of it happening time and time again. You may even have been guilty of it yourself. Every New Year people decide they will take more exercise and eat more healthily in an effort to lose weight. They become incredibly motivated in the gym and monitor every calorie that passes their lips for a couple of weeks. But when they do not see quick results or do not fully appreciate the results they have achieved so far, the automatic assumption is that exercise and healthy eating do not work and they give up completely, go back to their old routine and end up heavier than when they started.

Similarly, people enter sporting events or challenges to push themselves further than ever before and take their fitness to the next level. But they do not consider how their training programme needs to be progressive and they push themselves far too early into their training schedule, resulting in injury and less exercise than they managed previously.

The reality of the situation is that the human body takes a little time to adjust to new conditions. We are amazingly adaptable creatures, but you must give your body a chance. After many years of living with familiar exercise and food patterns, the body takes time to acknowledge that new patterns of behaviour and new ways of working are going to become the norm. If you keep up your new habits long enough for your body to recognize that the new routines are here to stay, you will soon reap the rewards. As the body adjusts to a new, increased level of exercise, your heart and lungs will become more efficient, your muscles and connective tissue will become stronger and you will burn more and more calories every time you exercise.

It is unfortunate but many people, having done the hardest part of starting a new regime, give up on it, just as their body is about to show them some positive results. Be patient and you will reap the rewards.

> Do you really want to achieve your aims, or would you like to end up worse than when you began?

If you were to say to someone embarking on a new fitness regime, 'would you like to achieve your aims, or would you like to end up worse than when you began?' they would think you were crazy. Of course they want to end up in a better situation otherwise they would not bother. But history shows that many people do end up in a worse situation and it is usually because they are unrealistic with the timing of their progress.

Take a moment and ask yourself which of the following two options you would rather have:

- Success with your goals in three months.
- Your old routine with its negative results back in place in two weeks.

You may be thinking you would rather have success with your goals in two weeks. So would everyone else. This is why they end up back where they started, or worse. If you are prepared to look beyond immediate rewards, take a different approach and look at the progress you could make during a one- to three-month period where you tackle your priorities in sequence, your task will be less daunting.

This longer-term view is beneficial because it allows you to make small, gradual and sustainable alterations to your routine over time. You do not have to fix everything at once so you can adopt a calmer, more thoughtful approach. You have a built-in margin of error for fact-finding and modifying your techniques along the way until you uncover what you need to do to achieve the results you want. You do not have to turn your life upside down in an attempt to achieve everything right now. You can take a more measured approach that will guarantee you get exactly where you want to be over the coming weeks, months and years.

Think about it again, guaranteed success in three months or guaranteed to be back where you started, or worse, in two weeks. Which would you rather have? It is time for you to take a new approach. Be different this time and be more successful than ever before!

The success equation

> **Fitness Pitfall 3:** Loss of motivation along the way
>
> **Usual Outcome:** Unfulfilling long-term success
>
> **The Road to Success:** The Success Equation

> Knowledge + Motivation + Timing = Success

One of the most striking things about us humans is what we are capable of when we turn our minds to something. This applies to everyone. We all have done and can do amazing things when we feel strongly enough. So far, we have highlighted how you can explore your fitness aims and ensure your goals are exciting and motivating. With something exciting to aim for and the right motivation, the drive to succeed and the creative thought around how to make our dreams come true can be unstoppable. So why can't we be unstoppable all the time? Why can't we make everything we want a reality? Why can't we get fitter when we want to, or shed pounds at will?

Our brains are fast and powerful and we are continually assessing the surroundings and how we fit into them. We are constantly on the lookout for signs that put us into context with where we are and who we are with. We are always pondering, 'how do I shape up to my environment and the individuals in it?' If, in our minds, we can place ourselves in an advantageous position in the environment, we feel good. If we sense that we do not match up in any way, our confidence can ebb away. It is this continual assessment of what is around us that leads us to ask ourselves if we need to change in any way. At times, we may consider how we might need to alter our mental attitudes, but usually we focus more readily on how we might need to change physically. How we look can become our primary concern.

When we think about what motivates us and what inspires us to change, we usually concentrate on a few simple factors. We think about how we currently live, our role in life, what we look like and how we feel. Often we tend to focus on all the negatives that exist in our lives and worry about what would happen if these negative factors were to grow beyond the current situation – what would life be like then and how would we cope with this?

We then consider what the alternatives are, what could be better than what we have, and how life would look and feel if we eradicated all the negatives and replaced them with more positive alternatives.

In a matter of a few seconds, our minds wander from a passing thought that someone we see looks good in an outfit, to being suddenly aware that a particular item of our own clothing does not feel as loose as it used to. From here we make a mental leap to a panic stricken, 'what if I'm putting on weight, what if all my clothes begin to feel tight, what if I never feel comfortable with these or any other clothes again?' Just as quickly, our thoughts turn to ways of avoiding these negatives, measures such as taking exercise or eating more healthily for a while. We know that taking these steps will help us control our weight, feel more comfortable in our clothes and allow us to feel that we are back in charge of ourselves and our position in society.

This is a typical and familiar process for most people. Thoughts like these are being filtered by your brain all the time. Sometimes they disappear as soon as they appeared as you get distracted by something else. Or, they may grow and you could be overwhelmed by them once a month, once a week or even several times a day, but the thoughts do not always lead us to change the way we behave.

Generally in life we follow pretty straightforward routines of behaviour and operate mainly within our comfort zone. On a day-to-day basis we do things that fulfil our needs and we try to keep ourselves as happy as possible. We may not always be completely satisfied with our lot but we learn to live with an acceptable level of dissatisfaction and discomfort which we tolerate as part of life's rich tapestry. In some cases, this discomfort is so familiar to us, it can even become a strong contributing factor to the comfort zone we inhabit.

It may be that you are not happy with your body shape but you have learnt to live with it. You can wear clothes that cover up a multitude of sins and in which you feel comfortable enough to go about your daily routine. You know that you could make some changes to your diet that would help you shed a few pounds and you understand that taking more exercise would make you feel a bit more lively, but you are getting by OK and you have got enough to think about, so why give yourself new things to worry about? There will be time in the future to make some changes here, but for the moment, your comfort zone is comfortable enough.

> Your trigger to motivation can come upon you at any time. Take full advantage of it when it does.

Then, one day, something happens that disturbs your comfort zone. Something that affects you more powerfully than ever before. It is usually one of two things. Perhaps something has triggered a negative thought about yourself that has spiralled out of control and become overwhelming. You become dissatisfied with your current situation in a way that you have never felt before. You feel upset and angry and you resolve that it is time to take action to fix things.

Alternatively you may be struck by something positive that you experience, you might see someone you admire and whom you would like to emulate. Or a particular event may trigger some positive feelings inside you. Having had a taste of this positivity you want to take steps to do more in life that will generate these feelings. Or you may be making plans for a future event that you are looking forward to, maybe a wedding, a holiday or a family visit. You can anticipate how good the event will be if you are in your peak mental and physical state so you decide to take action now to make sure this happens.

Positive and negative motivation

> What we have here are the two most common forms of motivation. The first is 'away from' or negative motivation, the other is 'towards' or positive motivation.

Negative motivation occurs where we either experience, or imagine, the worst case scenario for ourselves. With this experience or these thoughts inhabiting our minds, we feel strongly that we would do anything to change this situation for the better by moving away from where we find ourselves. Away from motivation can be triggered by the slightest change in perspective and can become effective overnight. It is the mental process that makes the person who has been three stone overweight for years, suddenly decide it is time to take action to lose some of the excess pounds. It is the same shift in mental attitude that can make a life-long couch potato suddenly go out and do something active.

Negative motivation is triggered at the precise point when the current situation is no longer tolerable and something must be done to move away from it right now. The motivation is strongest at this trigger point and can be sustained if translated immediately into action and results. The quicker the action taken and the results obtained, the more potent and long-lasting the motivation will be.

An important factor here is to resist the temptation to focus too much on how you arrived at your current situation as this can lead to restrictive thought patterns. Finding yourself in a situation that you feel desperate to move away from simply means that you have reached the right time to make things better, so embrace any uncomfortable feelings as part of the process of change and channel them into positive and creative thought processes to make things different from now on.

Positive motivation is a more controlled phenomenon. This is when we consciously create something positive in our mind around how we see ourselves in the future. We imagine where we want to get to, physically and mentally, very vividly, and we strive towards this image with great enthusiasm, making the changes to our lives that guarantee success. By creating a clear objective for the future we cultivate the motivation to take action to rapidly move towards our specific aims.

Both types of motivation are very powerful as inspiration to take action. Negative motivation usually finds us. It hits us when we have really had enough of how things are and feel we must do something about our current or anticipated negative situation. It is a strong call to action but can be limiting because, as soon as you have changed what you did not like, you may be inclined to halt your progress here.

Positive motivation is something we can act upon at any time simply by considering what would be more desirable and what we could do to improve on our current situation. Positive motivation has the edge on negative motivation when it comes to achieving results because of the natural feelings of progress that aiming towards your goals will bring you. Away from motivation can lead to a sense of relief when you make changes to your life and reach a better place. The powerful feelings of satisfaction and achievement that go with creating a positive future to move towards are much longer lasting than a short-lived sense of relief.

Away from motivation triggers	Towards motivation
Your trousers feel too tight	Going on holiday
You see something in your reflection that you really do not like	Attending a family/social event
Feeling repeated low energy	A romantic date
An observation or comment on your appearance from someone else	A sporting event
You feel you just cannot go on as you are any longer	Observing a role model living the life you would like to live

The strongest motivation can be evoked by a combination of away from and towards factors. Firstly, an away from trigger catches you suddenly and you feel you really must do something to change it. Before you make any knee-jerk reactions, sit down and think about what you want to work towards as well as what you want to move away from. Creating your fitness future in your mind and on paper satisfies all the criteria for successful change and is the most effective step you can take at this point. If your immediate reaction to an away from trigger is to throw out offending food or pack yourself off to the gym, there is a danger that your changes could be short lived. If you use the negative trigger as a call to plan what you are working towards, you will increase the likelihood that the action you take in your new plan is specifically geared to the most effective ways of achieving your goals. **From this point onwards, everything you do is directed towards the success you have created in your mind and this in turn leads to sustainable motivation.**

Take a moment now to think about what elements of your fitness you might like to move away from, and what you might like to move towards. What does ideal fitness look like to you? Can you picture clearly what you would like to move towards?

What elements of my current fitness do I want to move away from?	What is the fitness future that I want to move towards?

There is no need to be disheartened by noting down elements of your life that you are trying to get away from. This is simply a process of being honest about where you are currently. Sometimes it appears preferable to hide from the truth of the situation but this only creates obstacles on the road to success. Once you have honestly assessed and acknowledged the facts of the matter, you will be liberated to be creative with what you would prefer.

Spend most time on generating the full details of where you want to get to with your goals. Your motivation will be greater, fuller and longer lasting if you can create a crystal clear image of what you want and when you want it. Set yourself a complete challenge and detail everything that will be good about making this image a reality, and you will not stop until you have it.

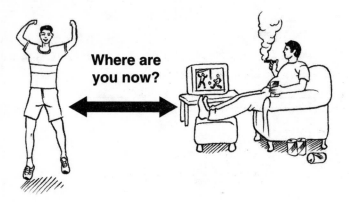

figure 1
where are you on the motivation equation?
what would have to happen in your life to move you in one direction or the other?
how far do you have to move in either direction to find your true motivation?

Maintaining motivation exercise

Having now given careful consideration to the details of what you are going to achieve in order to generate motivation, and having considered the different types of motivation that can create action, ask yourself the following questions. Answer honestly and frankly with as much information as possible and by the end of these three simple steps you will be ready to make changes. You have the motivation and the time is right for action. If there are any gaps in your 'how to' knowledge, these will be filled later in this book.

Step 1 The truth of the matter

The current situation with my fitness is ...

....

....

Step 2 Away from motivating triggers

If I continue as I am, the results will be ...

....

....

If my current patterns of behaviour become more extreme, the most negative consequences could be ...

....

....

Step 3 Towards motivating triggers

The most important things I want to achieve with my fitness are ...

....

....

If I make positive changes to my current fitness situation, the benefits will be ...

....

....

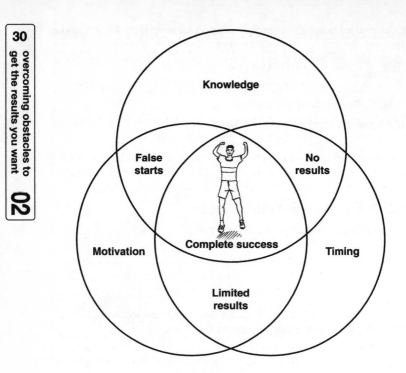

figure 2 knowledge, motivation and timing

Knowledge = what you need to do
Motivation = why you want to do it
Timing = when you will do it successfully

Knowledge + Motivation without correct Timing can lead to false starts with your fitness programme.

Motivation + Timing without Knowledge means your fitness plan will not be right for you and the results will be limited.

Knowledge + Timing without Motivation means no results.

Knowledge + Motivation + Timing = Success

Choosing the right fitness plan for you

Fitness Pitfall 4: Choosing an impossible plan

Usual Outcome: Feeling the task is too much and impossible to even begin

The Road to Success: Choosing the right fitness plan for you

Now that we have done some research into what you really want to achieve with your fitness and how to get motivated to take action, we need to examine how you are going to fit achieving these goals into your life, starting now.

Overcoming the fear of failure

Something that can discourage people from making changes to their lives is the fear that things might not work out just as they want them to. I once heard someone say, 'I do not like to fail at what I do so I would rather not put myself under too much pressure by going on a diet, just in case I cannot keep it up'. This is a great example of how creative we can be with our excuses to avoid what we know needs to be done. It shows how we can twist things in our own minds to suit what we want to believe at the time. Although this person was unhappy with their body shape and weight, they perceived that it was better to maintain the status quo than to take responsibility for making some changes. To set about making changes and not get the result they were looking for would lead to them being dissatisfied on two counts – in their mind they would be overweight *and* unable to take action to fix the situation. So they settle for just being overweight.

A significant reason that people anticipate 'failure' is that they expect to hit on the right solutions, the ideal fitness plan, immediately. What can we do to create a more positive vision of fitness where the notion of failure no longer exists?

From ideal to real

Most people love the idea of being a physically active, vibrant, sporty individual, taking exercise, eating well and living life to the full. So why is it that so many do not manage to live up to their ideals of what it means to be physically active? And, worse than that, having failed to live up to their ideals, why are people so hard on themselves for not doing 'enough'?

As you go about your daily routine in your office, on the train, in coffee shops or any social environment around the country, it won't be long before you hear someone bemoaning the fact that they should have gone to the gym last night and they feel really guilty because they now cannot go for another three days. Or that they broke their diet yesterday and they feel terrible because they just cannot seem to stick to eating the right things.

A common limitation for people embarking on a new fitness regime is that they do not stop to consider fitness, exercise and healthy eating within the parameters of their own lives. They read the latest books or magazine article, or see something on the television that discusses the 'perfect' answer or solution to healthy living, and all of a sudden they find themselves aiming for this perfection without considering whether or not it is appropriate for them. It looks quick and looks easy, so that is what they choose to aim for.

Everyone loves the idea of being healthier, fitter, slimmer or stronger but to be successful, each person must get into a position to become fully involved in what they want to achieve, how their lifestyle will allow them to achieve it and, crucially, by when. Only when these things have been considered, can you make your aims a priority, schedule your activities correctly and create an atmosphere of ongoing success to replace any notion of failure.

So, how do you know what your ideal fitness programme is? Firstly, ask yourself, 'if I achieved my ideal fitness, what would my life consist of and what would an average week of fitness look like?' The answers people can come up with here can be very ambitious with the ideal programme for an aspiring regular gym-goer often looking something similar to the schedule for an Olympic athlete.

So now ask yourself, 'when specifically will I be doing each part of my ideal schedule?' The ideas you come up with here will begin the process of turning your Olympian schedule into a more achievable proposition by focusing on what training you would like to do or would be able to do at different times on various days as you fit the programme together in your head. So far, so good.

Now comes the key question, which is often overlooked. Ask yourself, 'if this is my ideal schedule, with commitments to various activities at set times and days, would it work if I were to put it into action immediately?' Would it work if the week you are imagining in your head was this week? Would it work if you were to put it in the context of the other things going on in your life like work, family, friends, socializing and your other interests and hobbies? If not, what would work? Which of the elements of your 'ideal' fitness programme are really possible and even desirable given everything else that you have and that you enjoy in your life?

By acknowledging that your current ideal fitness programme could be an abstract ideal and not a realistic proposition for your current situation, you are now free to get on with designing a new schedule that can become your true ideal. This time, your ideal programme is designed specifically around your needs and your situation, it fits into your life, and is achievable.

Manage your expectations carefully. Aim too high and you will set yourself up for disappointment. Aim too low and progress will be slow. Think carefully about your ideal fitness programme and then slot it gently into your life.

Take time to create *your* ideal programme right now.

My Ideal Fitness Programme

If I achieved my ideal fitness, what would my life consist of?

....

....

What would an average week of fitness look like?

....

....

When specifically will I be doing each part of my ideal schedule?

....

....

If this is my ideal schedule, with commitments to various activities at set times and days, would it work if I were to put it into action immediately?

....

....

Which elements of my ideal fitness programme are possible in reality?

....

....

Everyone has the ability to plan a fitness programme they can easily follow and get results with. When you know your schedule you can plan when to put fitness into action and then you can forget about it for the rest of the time. So not only do you become the active exerciser you have always wanted to be, you will be liberated by success and free from the perpetual guilt of not living up to an ideal that was never realistic in the first place.

Injury and illness

Fitness Pitfall 5: Falling foul of injury or illness

Usual Outcome: An interrupted fitness plan leads to frustration and loss of routine

The Road to Success: Understand injury or illness and work around them

Embarking on a new fitness regime can be a daunting prospect if you are in good health and even more of a challenge if you are carrying a long-term injury or ongoing illness. If you have any kind of pre-existing medical condition at all you must seek advice from a doctor or a specialist before you put your fitness plans into action. There are two reasons for this. Firstly, you need to be medically safe to proceed and you must be sure that any action you take in a new regime is not going to aggravate your condition. Secondly, you need some initial guidance on what you will and will not be able to do. A medical specialist will provide you with early direction on what your programme should consist of to most effectively fix any long-term injury or work around any pre-existing medical condition.

If you develop an injury after you begin your new programme, seek advice on what you should do as soon as you can. Too many people are put off their exercise routine because of something quite minor that could be fixed in a matter of days. Letting a minor injury get in the way of fitness progress is often a sign there is something missing with the plan or the motivation and the injury is just a good excuse to avoid doing what needs to be done. Because your exercise plans have been so carefully considered, and your motivation is high, you will be in the opposite position and will be keen to fix any injury soon so you can get on with reaching your goals.

If you feel unwell but are not sure what is wrong, your GP should be the first person you visit. He will be able to diagnose your illness and advise you on the way forward, whether this be with medication or with an alternative solution. He/she will also be able to tell you whether or not it is wise to exercise prior to full recovery.

If you have injured yourself, your GP will advise you of what your specific injury is and how you can fix it. He/she may advise rest or he may advise specific exercises to correct a minor problem area. If your injury is more serious you will be referred to a specialist. This may be a physiotherapist, osteopath, chiropractor, podiatrist or any number of other experts, depending on your situation.

Top tip

Injury

This is simple advice. If you are injured and you visit your GP or an expert practitioner and they provide you with some rehabilitation exercises, **make sure you do them**. Many people allow a short-term injury to turn into long-term aggravation simply by not taking simple steps to fix the injury at an early stage.

Top tip

Illness

If you feel under the weather and you are not sure if you should exercise or not, use the following guidelines. If you are beginning to feel ill you may still be able to exercise but be careful. Go gently as your capacity for exercise will naturally be reduced as your body tries to fight off the illness. If you feel groggy above the neck and are suffering from cold symptoms, sore eyes or a runny nose, you are OK to exercise gently as long as you are safe and will not make your symptoms worse. If your bones are aching and you display symptoms of 'flu such as shivering or feeling hot and cold, you should rest until you feel better. Consider others when ill and do not go to the gym if you are in danger of passing anything on. As you recover you may be able to exercise outside with a walk, a gentle jog or bike ride and the fresh air could do you the power of good.

Success story – suddenly it all came together

If you still have reservations around the benefits of a more thoughtful approach to fitness success, here is an example of how precisely this approach was employed to overcome 20 years' worth of frustration and unhappiness.

Amanda had always been a picky eater with a sweet tooth. She stopped eating meat and chicken in her early twenties but other than that she never gave much thought to what she ate or why she was eating it. The result was that she ended up eating lots of carbohydrates as they were filling and convenient to prepare.

Amanda's weight had always fluctuated. When she was 17, she indulged in a variety of 'teenage crash dieting' and her weight dropped as low as 44.5 kg (7 st). At the time of her university graduation her weight crept up to 68.10 kg (10 st 10 lb). Her weight settled around the 63.5 kg (10 st) mark for the next 10 years, though Amanda admits to never being happy with this. When she got married, she dropped to 60.3 kg (9st 5 lb) through cutting down on carbohydrates and exercising with a combination of cardiovascular workouts and strength training.

Although Amanda was extremely dissatisfied with the way she looked, she never seemed quite able to get her weight under control. She just did not seem to have the time. For 17 years, work was always a higher priority as she focused on a fast-paced, highly stressed career with lots of travelling and client entertaining which played havoc with her food regime. She ended up eating lots of rich food at meal times in larger quantities than were necessary and then surviving on carbohydrates and sugar in between times in the hope this would keep up her energy levels.

The one thing that finally broke the cycle for Amanda was becoming pregnant. She was overjoyed to have two children within a couple of years but could not resist keeping a close eye on how this was affecting her weight, which fluctuated from under 63.5 kg (10 st) prior to her first pregnancy and peaking at just over 76 kg (12 st) during each of her pregnancies.

Following the birth of her second child, Amanda spent much of the next 18 months becoming increasingly more miserable with her body shape as her weight hovered once again around the 68 kg (10 st 10 lb) mark. She felt she had returned to where she was at her heaviest during her university days. During this period she took advice on exercise and through this managed to improve her fitness and strength levels. Something was still missing when it came to feeling motivated to make changes to what she was eating. Amanda was well aware of what she should do with regard to making simple changes to her diet, but never felt motivated to put these changes into practice.

Then, everything changed. A few cheeky comments about her shape from family members sparked a level of emotion that had not existed before. Amanda felt increasingly frustrated that she had got herself into a position where people felt they could comment, openly and negatively, on the way she looked. And one thing in particular marked the beginning of something new. Her three-year-old son pointed out some extra bits of flesh, 'Mummy's boobies on her back', which really depressed Amanda. She was disheartened to think that even her boy, one of the things she loved most in the world, had picked up on the fact that something was not as it should be with his mum and had pointed it out in a way that sent a message with the honesty and effectiveness that only a child could create.

At this point, it all came together for Amanda. She realized just how miserable she was with herself, but more than that she finally accepted that she just could not go on like this. She felt that from this moment onwards, she had no excuses for not fixing her situation.

She knew she had a good understanding of nutrition and what she should be eating, and she knew that she had all the information on exercise that anyone could ever need to make a difference to their body. She now felt there was no good reason why she should not be acting on what she knew. She decided there and then that it was up to her to just get on with it.

She thought about what had hindered her in the past. The main barrier to success that she could think of was that she always had unrealistic goals for herself, the favourite of which was to aim to lose 3 kg (7 lb) in a single week. Whenever she set herself this goal, she would start starving herself for as long as possible and by day four or five be driven by a frenzy to feast on chocolate, then be really fed up with herself, tell herself she had 'failed again' and vow to start again next Monday!

This time she was determined not to repeat the same mistakes of the past. She decided to start with a six-week plan, and drew up a schedule for the next six weeks on the calendar. The schedule contained all important dates such as a wedding anniversary and any special parties or occasions. She then set a goal of losing 7 kg (1 st) in six weeks. She broke this goal down even further so that she would be aiming to lose 2 kg (4 lb) in week one and then 1 kg (2 lb) during each subsequent week. Amanda decided she would weigh herself each Monday morning and if she had achieved her weekly goal, she would reward herself with a 'treat' which would be a new shirt, a belt, a manicure or some earrings – anything girly that made her feel she was succeeding would do the trick.

Amanda also forced herself to write down everything that she ate and drank every day in her food diary. She admits to thinking this tedious to begin with but then found it really useful to look back over each week, think about what she had consumed and how this had affected her energy levels on various days. She credits the food diary with teaching her how to examine her diet over a longer period and avoid the pitfalls of chocolate bars for the first time in her life.

The results were dramatic. Amanda managed to drop 7 kg (1 st) during her first six-week schedule. She then dropped an additional 3.5 kg (8 lb) with her second six-week plan. Buoyed by this success she went on to devise further six-week schedules designed to maintain her weight precisely where she had managed to get it and where she wanted it to stay.

For the first few weeks, Amanda was working through a back injury and so did a limited amount of exercise. From week four onwards she gradually increased her activity with a combination of running, strength training, yoga and hiking, usually managing some type of activity three or four times a week.

Amanda credits her success with not making changes to her diet that were too drastic. She cut out chocolate and reduced her wine consumption to a maximum of four glasses a week. By using her diary, she worked out that keeping off the carbohydrates after lunchtime, increasing her water consumption, and increasing her daily fruit and vegetable portions all worked extremely well and gave her the results she had always been looking for.

One of the biggest benefits that Amanda reports is that the great thing about where she is now is, apart from feeling lighter, fitter, healthier and happier, all of which are great on their own, she also feels 'empowered' with herself. She always secretly hated that word but now uses it to sum up the feeling of having taken charge and climbed one of her personal 'mountains'. Now she is so happy with her results and confident in her abilities, she is about to embark on targeting the next mountain, and this time it is a real one!

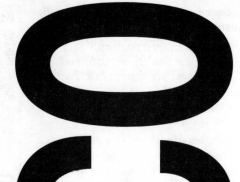

03

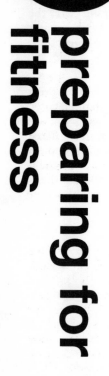

preparing for fitness

In this chapter you will learn:
- what kit you will need to get fit
- what equipment you will need to get fit
- everything you need to know on joining a gym and whether this is for you or not.

So now you have decided exactly what you want to achieve with your new fitness regime. You have your objectives, you have your motivation and the time is right for action. The next thing to do is to make sure you have all the resources you need to get going. There are a few vital items you need to give a little thought to:

- Clothing
- Footwear
- Equipment
- Training environment

Clothing

Make sure you have the right clothing for every type of exercise you will be doing. There is no need to spend a fortune on loads of fancy gear but you do need to be comfortable and you need to be supported in all the right places. Invest in the right underwear for your body shape, and some light clothing that allows you to move freely and keep cool. If you intend to exercise outdoors, having some waterproofs, or at least some items that protect you when it rains, will ensure you still take exercise when the weather is not being kind. Fitness is not fashion and you may not look as trendy as you might like in your workout gear, but there are some really great clothing lines for fitness on the market so you should be able to find gear that makes you feel confident as you exercise. And remember, with better fitness and a more toned body, you will look great in anything.

Footwear

Footwear is very important and worth spending a bit of time thinking about. Avoid choosing trainers just on looks and think instead about what you will be using them for. If you are intending to do a variety of exercise including visiting the gym and taking part in some classes, cross-trainers will be best for you. They can vary quite a lot in weight and in the shape of the shoe around your foot, particularly the height of the shoe around your ankle, so try on a few different pairs and move around in them to ensure you will be comfortable when exercising.

If you are intending to run as part of your programme, it is essential that you have the right running shoes for the way you walk and move. If you look around you will see how people can walk with very different styles. Some people walk with their toes turned out, some on the outside of their feet, some on the inside. The way they hold the top half of their body also affects how their feet make contact with the ground. To check how the way you walk impacts on your feet, take a look at a pair of shoes you use regularly and see how the soles are wearing.

If you walk particularly heavily on one part of your foot, chances are this effect will be exaggerated as you run. Landing awkwardly on your feet while running can lead to the rest of your body being out of its natural alignment. This in turn can lead to discomfort in your ankles, knees, hips, back and even shoulders and neck. At best, this discomfort might just be a distraction. At worst, you could end up with a long-term repetitive injury which will be painful and could hamper your fitness progress, or even put a stop to it altogether.

Take time at the beginning of your programme to visit a sports shop where they have the knowledge and experience to sell you trainers that suit the way you move. Some shops use a special electronic mat which you run across, allowing an image of your footprint or foot-strike to be seen on a computer screen. It is then clear to see where your weight is distributed as you run, and where you will require extra support from your trainers. More specialist running shops are staffed by experienced runners who can prescribe the best footwear for you simply by watching you in action.

There are an enormous number of shoes on the market and you should be able to find some that suit you. If you find that you just cannot find a pair that make your feet feel comfortable when you exercise, or you have persistent problems with your feet, you may need to visit a podiatrist who can examine your body alignment in more detail and, if necessary, design some extra supports to fit into your shoes. This may sounds extreme but ensuring your feet are supported properly is vital for successful exercise.

Equipment

I wonder what fitness equipment you have around your house at the moment. Maybe an old set of dumbbells, a skipping rope, some ankle weights, a mat, a bench or a fitball? And if you have this kit, is it ready for action? Has it been used recently?

It is an integral part of turning over a new leaf in your fitness regime. You plan what you want to achieve and then go out and buy the kit that will help you reach your goals. Then, for whatever reason, the kit does not get used. Maybe you do not know quite what exercises to do with it. You may be worried about getting it wrong and injuring yourself or perhaps you just do not have the space or the time for exercising at home. Then the weights gather dust, the exercise bike ends up with clothes strewn over it, and the multi-gym sits in the garage getting rusty.

Spending money on unnecessary fitness kit is frustrating and the equipment can end up haunting you and making you feel guilty for spending the money and not using it. All this can be prevented by asking yourself a few questions before you part with any cash.

- If I buy this piece of fitness equipment, what will I actually do with it?
- Where will I use this kit?
- Where will I store this kit?
- If I were to use this kit in the next seven days, when would I use it and what would I use it for?

If you cannot answer these questions quickly and easily, keep your money in your pocket. If you cannot think of what you would do with the kit, you need to do more research before you buy. You need to be able to visualize yourself putting your kit into action. Where will you be? In the bedroom, the living room, the garden? Can you imagine yourself using your kit around the house? If you cannot, chances are, you never will. You need to have somewhere handy you can store your kit. If possible it is good to get it out of sight so that your house still feels like a home and not a gym, but not so out of sight that it is out of mind as well. All home fitness kit should be hidden when you want it to be, and accessible when it is time to use it.

Finally, think about when you will be able to get started with your new kit. If you cannot find an opportunity to use it within the next seven days, the chances are that you will not be using it much beyond this first week.

Think carefully about the fitness programme you are about to embark on and what exactly you have decided it will consist of. Then you can clearly decide what kit, if any, you need to buy.

The options for exercising at home are endless and the main benefit is that you can create a time efficient workout regime with no travel time. With planning, a home fitness routine can be very effective. For more information on where to buy your kit, please refer to the fitness resources section at the end of the book.

Fitness facilities

It is a big decision – do you join the gym or not? Some people love them, some people hate them – which side of the fence do you fall on? Gyms and health clubs can be a fantastic motivator to exercise. They provide an enormous variety of equipment for you to choose from, all set up in an environment dedicated to getting fit. You have pleasant surroundings and a common goal with those around you, helping you to focus on your fitness without distraction. There are exercise specialists to consult on how best to use the equipment and how to get the most out of the time you spend exercising.

Health clubs also provide a selection of specialist classes where experts can guide you safely through new ways of exercising, and motivate you to exceptional results. Sampling a few different classes could help you discover a fresh style of exercise that really works for you, or give you options for a variety of workouts throughout the week that really keep you focused.

If you decide the gym is for you, there are a number of things to check before signing on the dotted line. You need to decide specifically what is important to you in a gym and then make sure that the gym you choose fits the bill completely.

Accessibility

Choose a gym that is easy for you to get to. If you are feeling in the mood for exercise, you will overcome all obstacles to ensure you get a workout but if you are feeling a bit tired or lacking in motivation, an awkward journey to the gym will be enough to put you off.

If you need to drive to the gym, check out the traffic on the route at various different times of the day and week. It may be all right if the journey takes five minutes on a Saturday morning, but what if it takes 30 minutes each way on a weekday evening? This just won't be practical in the long run.

Key criteria for choosing your gym	What to look out for
Accessibility	Where is it and how will you get there?
Environment	Are the setting, the building and the layout to your taste?
Opening hours	Do the hours suit your timetable? Is the gym open when you would consider using it?
Atmosphere	Do you get a good feeling when you are in the building?
Finances	Does this gym suit your budget and will you get good value for money?
Membership	Is there a membership package option that suits you?
Services	Does the gym offer all the services you are looking for? Do they have all the equipment that you would like to use?
Staff	Do the staff inspire you?

Make sure there is sufficient parking for everyone who is driving to the gym. Parking a little further away and then walking or jogging to the gym may not necessarily be a bad thing but it is better that you have the choice than being forced into it. Time spent looking around for parking spaces is bound to get frustrating eventually.

If getting to your gym involves a trip on public transport, is the route well serviced throughout the week? Ideally you want to be able to get to the gym easily whenever the mood takes you. Your journey should be safe, even if you do not finish your workout until the evening. You must also be comfortable on your journey. If the idea of travelling home on the bus or train feeling hot and sweaty after exercising does not appeal to you, you may end up avoiding gym visits completely, so consider things like this carefully in advance to prevent them from hampering your progress.

If you are lucky enough to find a gym close enough for you to walk, run or cycle to, you will be able to control your journey time as you travel under your own steam. Just make sure that your mode of travel suits you equally well all year round. If you enjoy the run or the bike ride to the gym in the summer, ask yourself honestly, whether the prospect will be so appealing when the weather is not so good. If you think cycling to the gym in the rain isn't you, make sure there is an alternative. It is fine to have different journey plans for the summer and the winter, just make sure when choosing your gym, that getting there is equally easy regardless of the season.

Environment

To ensure the best results, you need to be happy with every aspect of the environment of your gym. You need to be inspired by the look of it as you approach and you must be comfortable with the layout inside. Gym environments range from the remote country club with sweeping driveway, spacious gym, giant studios, juice bar, restaurant and social areas to smaller scale 'exercise only' options where sometimes even a changing area is seen as a bonus. On a very practical level, are the changing rooms clean and hygienic. Are the facilities air-conditioned, and does the air-conditioning work? This may not seem like a big consideration if you are joining a gym in January, but come the summer, you will wish you had checked. Ineffective cooling in the gym can make a workout very uncomfortable, or worse put you at risk of overheating or dehydrating. Choose the environment that suits your needs and that you feel most comfortable in. Check out a variety of different size facilities and choose the one you can most clearly imagine yourself physically inside, walking around and working out in.

Opening hours

Most health clubs appreciate that the majority of people need to exercise either before or after work and their opening hours reflect this. Many open at 6.00 a.m. or 6.30 a.m. and will stay open until 10.00 p.m. or 10.30 p.m.. There are even some 24-hour gyms springing up to make working out accessible for everyone, no matter what their working pattern or lifestyle. There are still some facilities that open for shorter hours, for example some local council services are only open from 9.00 a.m. to 6.00 p.m. so take care to check that your gym will be open when you want it to be.

Atmosphere

Your gym has to have an atmosphere that suits you. The look and layout of the building is one thing, the feelings that you get from the place are another thing entirely. Does the gym exude a no-nonsense approach to getting fast results or does it feel more gentle and supportive? Which are you most comfortable with? Consider what kind of atmosphere is going to draw you to the gym, even when you might not feel very enthusiastic, and will encourage you to get the most out of your exercise.

Finances

Money is always a consideration when joining a gym, but rather than focusing on the amount that you will be spending, think about what you will be getting for the money. Where are you going to get the best value for money? Obviously, you cannot buy fitness, but you can invest your money wisely to ensure you get results with your fitness programme. You can join a gym for a relatively small amount of money these days, just be sure it is a gym you are happy to go to regularly.

Rather than focusing on the regular monthly fee for a health club, think about how much each visit will work out costing you. A relatively low monthly membership ends up looking expensive if you manage only one visit every three weeks because you do not like the gym. If you feel you need to spend a little more to get membership to a gym or health club that offers a little extra, and this little bit extra will encourage you to get there more often, think about how this affects the cost per visit. If the monthly fee is slightly higher but you visit the gym twice a week then you will certainly be getting more value for money out of your membership.

Money is a consideration but it should not be a barrier to joining a gym. Focus on what you will get from your gym membership rather than what you will pay for it, and you will think of all sorts of ways to come up with the money. You could probably save the amount you need each month by giving up a few visits to the coffee shop or passing up on a couple of nights out.

Membership

Make sure you investigate exactly what you will be signing up for. You need to know how much you will be paying and how often. Most health clubs charge a joining fee and a monthly membership. More often than not, the monthly membership is for a minimum of 12 months with a notice period following that of one to three months. You need to be happy signing up for a minimum of a year. Because you have planned carefully what you want to achieve with your fitness programme, you will know precisely how you are going to be spending your time in the gym during this first year, and beyond, so the decision should be clear. There is no need to be concerned about working on your fitness for at least 12 months to come; the only thing to clarify is whether this health club is the one for you and whether their membership structure will support you in your aims.

Many health clubs will offer you a day pass or maybe even a free weekly trial so you can check out the facilities. If they do not offer it, you must ask. Having a tour around a gym or health club is one thing but it is no substitute for testing it out properly. A trial day or weekly membership will allow you to try out your journey and sample what it is like to approach the gym, go through reception, get changed, have your workout, shower, maybe have a drink or snack, healthy of course, a chat with the staff or other members and then make the journey home. Only when you have tried all of these things can you make a decision on whether the routine works for you or not, and if you decide that it does not quite suit you, you do not want to have to wait a year or more to be able to try something different. You are not being demanding by asking to test things out, just being thorough. Health clubs should welcome your diligent research as this will make you a more committed member when you do join. Any gym that will not allow you to try out their facilities should not really be given much more consideration.

There are gyms that offer shorter rolling contracts or pay-as-you-go systems. This is often a more acceptable way of proceeding as it allows flexibility to change your approach whenever you want to. You may think it is a sign of your commitment to yourself that you are signing a 12 month contract to work on your programme but be cautious with this line of thinking. If your choice of fitness venue turns out not to provide all that you hoped it would, you may be in danger of not going and then losing momentum with your fitness programme altogether. If you have the flexibility to alter the venue whilst keeping your programme in place, you are more likely to continue to make positive progress.

Services

It is vital to clarify what your membership includes. If you are intending to use the gym, make sure the membership includes an initial programme and regular reviews and updates of how you are spending your exercise time. With the help of this book, you will be fully equipped to design your own fitness programme and progress it over time but there is no harm in seeking further information if it is there on tap. Regular checks on how you are proceeding will assist you with your results and any gym worth its salt should insist on checking up on how you are doing.

Walk around the whole gym area and see what equipment is there. Look out for your favourite bits of kit to make sure you can find them. If there is equipment you are not familiar with, find out what it does and if it will be of interest to you and your objectives. If the equipment looks complicated, find out how it works by asking for a demonstration. Check everything is well maintained and safe. Modern, clean equipment that's kept well is a sign that the gym and the people in it are being managed well and take pride in what they do.

Establish whether or not all classes are included in your membership fee. These days, most gym chains will include classes with the membership but it is worth checking just to ensure that the classes you may be joining up specifically to attend do not end up costing you extra.

If you are interested in attending classes, ask to see a timetable of when each class takes place. You need to make sure the classes are running when it is convenient for you to get to them and you need to find out how busy they are. If you can only attend classes at peak times, make sure there will be room for you. Ask someone at the gym how busy the classes get or, better still, drop by when the class you want is running and take a look at how many people are in it. Find out if you need to book your classes in advance or if you can just turn up. It is important to know as there is nothing worse than making the effort to get to the class only to find out that you forgot to book your place. If it is necessary to book, and bookings work on a first come, first served basis, can you guarantee you will always be able to get your name down quickly enough?

In addition to the gym area and the traditional exercise classes, is there anything else you are looking for in a gym? Would you like to try yoga or Pilates as part of your weekly fitness routine? Do they offer other services such as a running club, cycling club, netball or football club? Do they organize extra events that you might be interested in such as workshops or seminars on new approaches to exercise, nutrition, and other lifestyle themes? Do they organize social events and, if they do, what kind of events? Could your gym open up a world of opportunities for you as well as being the place to help you get in shape?

Staff

A good gym will be staffed by good people. Before you sign up, think about your experience of every person you come into contact with. Did you have a good feeling when made your first call to the gym? Were you received well when you arrived for the first time? How do the staff look? Are they smartly turned out with an enthusiastic air about them? Do they acknowledge you as you would wish them to, and do they inspire you to join their world?

Ask as many questions as you can of as many people as possible before making your final decision to join. If you get the impression that a particular health club is a good place to work, chances are it will be a good place to work out. Talk to the gym staff as these will be the people advising you on your programme, your technique and your regular updates. Ask them about their qualifications and how their education will help you. Ask them specific questions based on what you are going to achieve at the gym and listen carefully to their responses. Make sure you feel comfortable with them and confident in their abilities. Good gym staff should be confident in their technical ability and able to communicate their knowledge effectively.

Speak to the people who teach the classes, particularly the classes you are interested in and find out if you have a good rapport with them. You do not want to end up in a class where you do not like the instructor's methods, and you will not go back after the first class, so find out who will be leading your classes at the earliest opportunity.

Finally, talk to existing members and ask their opinion of the facility. Find out what made them join, has the gym lived up to their expectations, has it over-delivered or are they disappointed in some way? What are they most happy or most unhappy with? Are they glad they joined and are they still happy to be a member?

Where will you exercise?

There is much to consider when planning your fitness routine, and the choice of where you will exercise can be crucial. Here are a few things to look out for when making your decision.

I should join the gym	• It is a dedicated exercise environment.
	• There are other people around to help with motivation.
	• There is access to a variety of fitness options.
	• There is a good social scene
I should exercise at home	• No travel time involved.
	• I like to exercise outside
	• I would save money by not paying a gym membership.

What works for you?

Now you have chosen your venue for exercise, you can begin your programme and start getting results.

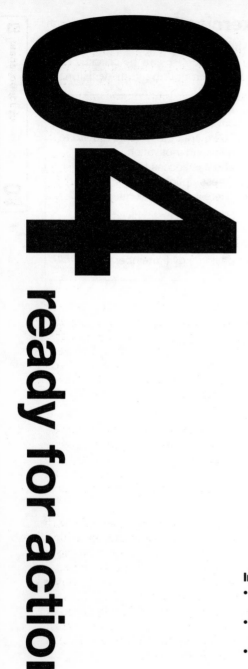

04

ready for action

In this chapter you will learn:
- how to compile a food diary and an exercise diary
- what to look out for with your diaries
- how to use the diaries to shape your future.

Once you have decided whether you would prefer to exercise at home or at a health club, the first thing to do is to gather information on what exactly is going on with your current routine – your exercise, food and lifestyle. People struggle with getting the right results with their fitness plan for one of two reasons. Either they do not alter their current routine enough to make any noticeable difference to how they look and feel, or they make too many changes all in a short space of time, upsetting their routine beyond what they are comfortable with and therefore beyond what they can sustain. With the latter situation, even if some positive results are achieved, you are never quite sure which of the changes led to the most positive results and your recipe for success can remain a bit of a guessing game.

> At any given time, you know the results of your current lifestyle and approach to food and exercise because you are living with them.

The most effective way to achieve the quickest change in these results is to examine your lifestyle in detail, analyse your regular habits and how you are behaving, and draw out the elements that are simple to change and that you can monitor. You need to know specifically what is working well for you already so you can do more of it. If something is not working so well for you, you need to be aware of this quickly so you can try something else.

The easiest way to monitor your behaviour is to keep diaries. Logging all of your weekly physical activities and dietary habits in an exercise diary and a food diary will tell you everything you need to know about where you are now with your fitness, and what changes you can make quickly and easily for the most effective results.

Writing things down encourages you to engage mentally with everything you do. By making some behaviours that may have become unconscious over the years into more conscious activities, you will be re-educating yourself as to the benefits, or otherwise, of what you are doing. A common example of this is found with food or drink. If you examine a typical day's or week's food and drink, you can probably highlight some behaviour patterns that have, over the years, become regular habits, such as a daily coffee on the way to work or a couple of biscuits each day as your mid-afternoon snack.

These habits are generally unconscious and are perpetuated because they become familiar and comforting and need no mental engagement. You do them because you always have. By writing down the coffees or the biscuits every time you have them, you are bringing the habits back into conscious thought and into the part of the brain that will begin to question your own behaviour and its consequences.

Once a habit becomes more conscious, it can be analysed within the context of the question, 'is this behaviour helping me to achieve what I set out to achieve, or is it hindering my progress instead?' When you begin to question yourself in this way you will very quickly see how you can make small daily changes that will dramatically quicken your progress. If you have herbal tea or water instead of each of the coffees, how might that impact on your energy levels? If you have fruit or some nuts instead of the daily biscuits, what type of extra nutrients would you be filling your body with and how many excess calories would you avoid over the course of a week?

> It is in the moments when we pause for thought that the battle for our health, fitness and nutrition goals is won or lost.

If you plan a weekly exercise schedule and then implement it without thought or hesitation, chances are you will complete everything you set out to do. If you stop along the way to give your schedule too much further consideration, you will probably talk yourself out of it. The same is true with food and our healthy eating plans. The quickest way to formulate your personal plan for success is to monitor everything you do and gradually amend your approach until you establish a way that works.

You will get incredibly positive feelings from writing down your achievements in your diaries and looking back over the good things that you have done each day and week. Keeping exercise diaries and food diaries encourages you to stick to your schedule because, having felt these positive feelings, you can anticipate feeling them again and you know what to do to make sure this happens. You will also want to avoid having to write down any excuses for missing a training session or making notes on the things you have eaten that were not so good, and this will help you stick to what you know will ensure you achieve your goals.

Sometimes people shy away from the idea of keeping food and exercise diaries and this is often a good indicator of just how unhappy they are with their current situation. In this situation, the diaries work brilliantly. Even if you think what you note down will be terrible to begin with, the idea is to collect the evidence of what leads to the current unsatisfactory results. This enables you to spot the simple changes that can be made to lead to improvement. No one needs to see your diaries. The very act of writing will help you to focus on what you are doing and, over time, the full picture will emerge and you can focus on the process of assessing your situation and making the changes you need to.

The diaries help you to generate your own positive behaviour change. We know there are thousands of books and exercise programmes out there. Using the diaries is a way of devising your own personal diet and exercise plan. You can use other resources to research what changes you could be making and the diaries will show you how realistic and effective these changes really are for you. Knowing this, you can adjust your choices accordingly.

Keeping food and exercise diaries is a simple technique that can lead to dramatic results. If you need any further evidence of this, try it yourself and see how keeping accurate records in these areas helps you to focus on what you do and whether your current behaviour is helping you with your goals or hampering your progress towards them.

Let's look at an example.

Sample weekly exercise/activity diary

To give you the full picture of your current exercise behaviour and its results, note down all exercise/activity for each week. Also make a note of how motivated you felt, how much you enjoyed the exercise and any other observations you may have on each workout.

Motivation

Rate your motivation level out of ten. Zero out of ten for motivation means you really did not feel like doing it, ten out of ten means that you were really excited/looking forward to your activity.

Enjoyment level

Rate your enjoyment level out of ten. Zero out of ten for enjoyment means that at no point during the activity, or afterwards, did you feel it was enjoyable. Ten out of ten means you enjoyed the activity to the maximum.

Day/Date	Time	Exercise/ Activity	Motivation Level (0–10)	Enjoyment Level (0–10)	Mood/ Thoughts/ Observations
Mon 8 Nov	7.30 a.m.	Walked the dog; 25 minutes walking for commute to work			
Tues 9 Nov	Morning and evening	Walking – dog and commute			
	7.15 p.m.	30-minute bike ride	3	7	It was cold and I did not fancy it but it was OK when I got going.
Wed 10 Nov	Morning and evening	Walking – dog and commute			
Thurs 11 Nov	7.45 p.m.	Weights session at the gym followed by a swim	7	4	I really felt like I needed to go to take my mind off everything I had done today but I felt tired when I got going and didn't really enjoy it.
Fri 12 Nov	Morning and evening	Walking – dog and commute Lots of meetings out of the office today so a lot of walking between them			
Sat 13 Nov	8.00 a.m 10.30 a.m.	Walked the dog Netball	5	9	Great to see my friends and have a run-around too.
Sun 14 Nov	11.00 a.m.	90-minute walk	6	7	Nice day, walking cleared my mind.

What do diaries tell us?

The longer the period you keep your diaries for, the more accurate a picture you will create of your behaviour and its consequences. Keeping the diaries for seven days should give you a useful snapshot of what is going on.

What to look for with your exercise diary

Writing down all exercise and activity that you do in a week illustrates very clearly a major part of the behaviour that brings you your current fitness level, body shape, energy levels and body fat content. Put very simply, if you continue with this level of activity, you will maintain your current state of fitness. If you do less than you do now, your fitness levels will decrease, if you do more, you will see improvements.

The human body is very efficient and will adapt itself to the surrounding conditions in order to protect us and make life easy for us. If we eat more than we need, our body assumes we are stocking up for a forthcoming food shortage and so it packs on body fat wherever it can so it can use it as energy in the future. If we exercise regularly, our bodies become conditioned to using fat as a source of energy. Thankfully, our bodies are very adaptable and we can easily make the change from one way of being to the other.

Our bodies respond to change and overload. Do what you have always done and your body will remain as it is. Do a bit more, something tougher, something a bit different and you will see different results. Monitor these results with your diary to pinpoint what works best for you and what works quickest. This will lead you to your optimum fitness plan for your specific aims.

Use your diary to find out specifically what is happening right now. Whatever you can add to this will make some kind of difference, so what *should* you add in order to make the changes that you want to see?

Exercise kick-starts your metabolism. Raising your metabolic rate burns fat calories. Regular, ongoing exercise speeds up your metabolism permanently meaning you become a more effective fat burning machine, every day and every night.

Sample daily food diary

To give you the full picture of your current eating behaviour and its results, note down everything you eat, when you eat it, how hungry you were at the time, and how you felt before, during and after each meal, snack or drink.

For the hunger rating, zero means you were full and were not hungry at all but were eating simply because food was there, you were bored, or there was some other reason to eat. Ten out of ten indicates that you were starving and ready to eat anything! For most times when you eat you will be somewhere between the two ends of the scale.

Example Day

Day/Date/ Time	Food/Meal/ Drink	Hunger Rating (0-10)	Moods/Thoughts/ Observations
Mon 8 November			
10.30 a.m.	Coffee and muffin	10	Monday morning, terrible journey to work, needed something comforting
11.00 a.m.	Glass of water		
1.30 p.m.	Chicken sandwich crisps, apple	6	My usual lunch, enjoyed it, felt good afterwards
2.30 p.m. & 6.00 p.m.	Glass of water		
3.30 p.m.	Cup of tea and two biscuits	7	Felt a bit tired so had something to pep me up
9.30 p.m.	Two glasses of wine Pasta, chicken, pesto sauce, bit of salad. Cheesecake	10	Finished work late so felt a bit rushed but happy that I managed to knock this meal together despite it being quite late
11.00 p.m.	Cup of tea	1	Need my bedtime cuppa

What to look out for with your food diary

Timing and quantity

When you eat is every bit as important as *what* you eat. Energy is stored in two areas in your body – in your muscles as glycogen and as fat in various areas around the body. The body's capacity to store energy in muscles is limited while our capacity to store fat is, as you will know all too well from some of the obese people you may have witnessed, almost endless. When we eat, we top up the levels of energy in our muscles and we can, if we eat the wrong food or too much food, add to our fat stores.

If you leave long gaps between meals your blood sugar levels will drop, your appetite will increase and you will feel hungry. This situation creates two danger zones. Firstly, because your blood sugar is low, your instinct will be to stabilize it as soon as possible and your body will begin to crave quick-fix sugary snacks. The second danger zone is that, because you are hungry you are likely to eat quickly leading to poor digestion and overeating. It takes around 20 minutes for the brain to register that the stomach is full so you need to eat slowly to allow your body to register when you are full and when you should stop eating. If you are over hungry and eating too fast, there is a danger that you could spend the 20 minutes it takes for the full signals to move around your body loading up with extra calories. Wait another 20 minutes and you will be feeling horribly bloated and full.

Eating small meals regularly keeps your blood sugar within comfortable levels and allows you to make sensible choices over what you eat. By not being over hungry at any given time the size of your meals will be reduced, meaning you take in an amount of calories appropriate to how many calories you need for fuelling your body for your daily routine. Consuming the right amount of calories through making positive food choices means there are no excess calories being stored as increased body fat.

Eat little and often and never go for more than four hours without food.

Food Myth 1

By eating less, my body will have to take energy from fat around my body and I'll lose weight.

This theory falls down on two counts. If you do not eat regularly you will starve your muscles of energy or glycogen. Without the presence of muscle glycogen, it is difficult for your body to burn fat. Also, if you do not eat regularly your body will assume there is a food shortage and will switch to fat-saving mode – the opposite of the situation you are trying to create. For the most effective fat burning you need to eat sensibly and eat regularly.

Hydration

The signals sent to your brain when you feel hungry are very similar to the signals sent when you feel thirsty. It is possible to reduce your overall calorie intake during a day by taking a drink when you first experience these feelings. A glass of water or fresh fruit juice, or a cup of mint or camomile tea may be all you need at that time. Drinking frequently between your meals and snacks can prevent any unplanned and unwanted calories being eaten and stored as fat.

Being properly hydrated also enables your body to work efficiently and carry out all of its functions as effectively as possible. This includes digesting food and burning calories so if you are aiming to lose weight, you need to be hydrated at all times.

If you feel thirsty, you are very probably already dehydrated so get some water immediately and begin sipping it regularly. For our busy modern lives, availability of water at all times is one of the main concerns for everyone looking to stay hydrated. Accessibility is the key and this comes only with forward planning. You need to look carefully at your daily and weekly schedule and consider where you will get your water on the go. If you work in an office, is there a water cooler you have easy access to where you can fill up your glass regularly? If there is, make sure you use it. If there is no water cooler, you will need to make sure you have enough water of your own to get you through each day.

If you are out on the road, plan where you can stop for water and also where you will be able to stop to use the toilet. The benefits of good hydration can be overshadowed if you end up desperate for the loo and find yourself with nowhere to go. If you are increasing your regular water intake, do it gradually and your body will get used to dealing with the extra fluid naturally and you should not get caught short. Keeping track of your fluid intake and its effects with your diary will highlight your optimum intake for hydration and comfort.

Food Myth 2

All liquids are created equally.

We have an enormous variety of drinks to choose from these days. Coffee now comes in a multitude of forms with all sorts of extras and there is an even greater variety of teas on the market. We have fruit juices, fizzy drinks, sports drinks, energy drinks, milk, milkshakes, yoghurt drinks and smoothies. And we have water. If you are aiming for optimum hydration, water is the best drink for you. The others have their individual attributes; coffee can temporarily pep you up, energy drinks can boost your performance and smoothies are a great way to get some extra nutrients into your body.

You must always be aware of what goes with each of your choices of drink. Coffee and fizzy drinks contain caffeine which acts as a diuretic and can lead to overall fluid loss. Fruit juices can be quite concentrated and digesting them can actually remove water from your system. Energy drinks can be quite heavy on sugar and calories, and smoothies may contain artificial additives. They can all have their place in your weekly food routine as long as you maintain an awareness of the benefits and otherwise of all liquids that you put into your body. Your aim is to be well hydrated and drinking the right amount of water for you is the quickest way to achieve this. Make this your priority and fit in other drinks where appropriate.

Top tip

Make as much of a fuss over your drinks of water as you do over other drinks. We often make a ritual out of preparing coffee, tea or a nice glass of wine but give little thought to how we drink water. Create a positive experience around water by making sure it is the right temperature for your taste, add ice if necessary and add a slice of lemon or lime to give it a little flavour. Make it a drink you can enjoy, not just a necessary evil.

Habits

Your food diary will show you everything that you eat and drink because you have formed habits around these items. Using the diaries we can question whether these habits work well for us or not. Popping to the kitchen to make a quick cup of tea can become a familiar routine whenever you have a quiet moment, but how many cups of tea do you really need in a day? And how many cups do you actually want? The strange thing about habits is that they sometimes lead us into behaviour that does not sit comfortably. You find yourself making yet another cup of tea even though you do not really want it but, because you have made it, you drink it anyway.

The same thing is true with snacks, cakes, biscuits, crisps or chocolate. None of these items is unquestionably 'bad' but what makes them bad for us is the quantity that we eat. They can all feature in your weekly intake but make a conscious decision on how much and how often. One or two desserts during a week may not do you too much harm, but if you fall into the habit of taking dessert after every meal, you can encounter problems with your calorie intake and your energy levels.

This is where the hunger rating scale on your food diary comes in. We fall into habits so that we do not have to think about every single thing we do. These patterns of behaviour can become extreme when people fall into the habit of having the same meal at the same time every day. This is quite common with breakfast, for example. Most people are too tired or too busy sorting themselves and their family out for the day to be creative with their breakfast choices. We stick with what we know and often eat it as quickly as we can.

Habitual choices at lunchtime are also quite common. This is sometimes down to time and sometimes down to accessibility. If you are busy at work, it is easiest just to grab the usual sandwich and get back to what you were doing. Problems arise when people fall into extreme habits of eating the same things at each mealtime every day. These are the people who love routine and love familiarity but they may not love the effects these comfortable routines and habits have on their bodies.

The hunger scale is effective for breaking habits. It can highlight the times you eat when you are not really very hungry. This is a very common situation when we are stuck in familiar eating habits. If you are used to eating the same things at the same times, you may not even be hungry when you are taking those meals. Eating when you are not hungry is likely to lead to weight gain and so should be avoided at all costs. Establishing just how hungry you actually are will enable you to eat according to your body's needs. This will help you establish whether or not you need to change the habits that you have developed and, if you do, what new tactics you can employ to get a better result.

Similarly, if your eating habits leave you starving before each meal, you are very likely to overeat leading to a similar result – you will gain weight. If your hunger rating is nine or ten out of ten before every meal, you need to think about altering your meals to incorporate some longer-lasting energy sources or inserting some healthy snacks between meals to help you feel a bit fuller more often.

Energy levels

All meals and food products fall into one of two classifications; food that gives us energy and food that robs us of energy. Put very simply, we need to increase the amount of food we eat that gives us energy and eliminate the products that rob us of energy. But how do we know which is which?

Completing the 'mood/thought/observation' column of your food diary is vital for monitoring why you make particular food choices and then whether or not the choices you made actually lived up to expectations. If you opted for a coffee and a muffin to pep you up, did it actually work? If you chose a pasta dish over a pizza because you wanted to feel less bloated, did this turn out to be the case?

An important question to ask yourself when thinking about food in relation to energy levels, is 'what is actually in this product and in what way will the contents provide me with energy or rob me of energy?'

As a guideline for making food choices, think about human evolution. Mankind evolved by living on the natural foods it could find, when it could find them. Cavemen and women ate what grew in nature and they ate little and often. Our bodies have changed very little from this period and are still designed to eat in this way so think about this as you make your decisions on food. If it is natural and grown, chances are we will have the capabilities to digest it relatively easily and to use the nutrients the food provides us with effectively in our bodies. If it is man-made, processed, refined, manufactured or artificially preserved, our bodies have a lot of work to do to break down and digest the unnatural products before we can get to the goodness of these foods, if in fact they have much goodness in them.

Natural foods contain a whole range of vitamins and minerals that are vital for our bodies to work to the best effect. They are essential to nourish the body and to enable all the chemical reactions necessary for life within the body to take place. If we consume these nutrients we feel vibrant and energetic. In the absence of these nutrients and with the inability of the body to perform some of the functions the nutrients are necessary for, we feel sluggish and below par.

Your food diary will be the most effective tool you have for monitoring where you can substitute energy robbers with energy-giving food products. You can then refine the process to look at where, when and how you can provide yourself with the best energy possible for achieving your fitness aims.

Something else you will notice from your food diary is how the quantity of food that you eat can affect your energy levels. If you are hungry you tend to eat more in the hope that you will restore your energy levels to normal but use your diary to see whether or not this is actually the case.

Eating to restore blood sugar levels is the right thing to do but eating relatively sweet foods and overeating can lead to lower energy and lower blood sugar levels than when you began. When you ingest food into your blood stream, your blood sugar will rise, but if it rises too quickly or too far, your body will begin to produce insulin to regulate your blood sugar. A rapid rise in blood sugar will lead to rapid production of insulin which may lead to an overall drop in blood sugar and energy levels.

This thinking forms the basis of the Glycaemic Index (GI). The index is a rating system with pure sugar at the top, scored as 100 on the index. Pure sugar is the food product that is absorbed fastest into the blood stream as its absorption is unimpeded by the presence of any vitamins, minerals or nutrients. Products beneath sugar on the index contain differing amounts of elements that enable the body to digest them more slowly and so they have a lower rating on the index. For example, some fruits contain sugar so you may expect them to be high on the index but the presence of fibre enables your body to absorb the sugars more slowly and lower the score of these items on the GI. Natural carbohydrates such as potatoes and vegetables are lower on the index than refined carbohydrates like pasta and white rice. Protein is low on the index and can be used to lower the index rating of an entire meal – a meal containing pasta and tomato sauce will have a higher rating on the index than the same meal which includes some chicken or fish.

Top tip

If your salad does not do the trick at lunchtime, try adding some protein to create a slower energy release meal. Cheese is an option for protein but does contain a relatively large amount of fat. Better than this would be to add some beans or pulses or some low fat meat such as fish or chicken.

So how does the glycaemic index help us with our energy levels? If you suffer from low energy and your diary shows you why this might be, looking to the glycaemic index for inspiration on alternative food choices will be a very effective way of improving your energy balance.

Top tip

When looking to improve your energy balance, try simple changes first. If a fruit snack does not fill you up for long, try a handful of nuts and seeds. These contain a little more fat than fruit but it is the good fat that the body needs and it helps you to feel full for a little longer.

Variety

Your diary will clearly show you how much variety you have in your weekly food and drink intake. Different foods contain different nutrients which help our bodies to work effectively. Your objective is to get as much variety into your food diary as possible. Select foods with different colours, textures and consistency whenever possible and use your diary to establish which combination works best for you and gets you the best results.

Alcohol

We could not write a section on examining what you eat and drink without giving proper attention to alcohol. For most of us keeping a food diary for around a week, alcohol will make an appearance at least once. It is a more regular feature for some than for others. We would not presume to make judgements on how much people like to drink but your weekly and monthly alcohol intake is an important consideration when considering your fitness and your figure.

Most people are familiar with the possible negative long-term consequences of alcohol, and we all hope they will never be a consideration for us. Heart disease, liver and kidney problems, obesity and depression are not things we are likely to want to envisage in our future. But what about the short-term implications of using alcohol in relation to our overall fitness and, in particular, our fitness for everyday life?

Alcohol is an important factor because it can play a part in each one of the areas we need to watch out for when analysing our food diaries. It can influence the timing of our meals and the size of these meals, and it can affect our hydration levels. It can become a habit that works against us rather than to our advantage and it can dictate our energy levels. It can also influence the decisions we make on the variety of food that we eat.

Timing

If you are not careful, alcohol can wreak havoc with the timing of your meals. The problem seems to occur most often in the early evening of some weekdays. As the clock approaches five, six or seven o'clock, you have had a long day and you have been working hard. It has been a while since your afternoon snack and even longer since you had something more substantial at lunchtime so you are beginning to feel a bit peckish. But because you are tired and because you deserve to relax and unwind a bit, pouring a nice glass of wine is far more appealing than getting started with the evening meal preparations.

The wine is also appealing because it contains fast-releasing energy so it will take the edge off your building hunger. The downside of this is that, by blunting the hunger temporarily with relaxing but nutrient-poor alcohol, you are prolonging the period when your body has to exist without nutrient-rich food. You will be in danger of entering the 'more than four-hours without eating properly' danger zone where your body will begin to think that it needs to slow your metabolism and store calories.

If you do have a drink some evenings to unwind, ensure that you eat something pretty soon after your drink and do not allow your enjoyment of the alcohol to cause you to skip meals until hours later or maybe even miss a meal completely.

Hydration

Alcohol is a diuretic so whenever you drink you need to make up for the fluid that you will lose. Fluid loss and dehydration mean that you will suffer the next morning.

A simple strategy to achieve this is to alternate your drinks with water – one glass of wine, one glass of water, or even two glasses of wine and then some water. Your diary will help you isolate what quantity of alcohol 'works' for you. you will clearly be able to see when you drink and enjoy it, and when you drink and it is not enjoyable. Be honest with yourself about how much alcohol you need or want. One glass may be lovely, a second glass still enjoyable but do you really want the third and the fourth. Are you having these because you are still savouring the drink or simply because you have established the pattern for the evening and are sticking to it? There comes a point in most evenings where we just focus on the action of drinking and what is in the glass can become almost irrelevant. Use the feedback from your diary to establish at what point you should make the switch from dehydrating yourself to rehydrating yourself. You will be thankful in the morning that you did.

Habits

Drinking alcohol is often referred to as habitual behaviour. Habits are behaviour patterns that we carry out without thinking and drinking certainly falls into this category in our modern culture. Alcohol has become synonymous with and associated with a variety of events and with the full range of emotions. We drink at weddings, we drink at funerals, we drink to celebrate, we drink to commiserate, we drink as part of a build-up to a night out, and we drink to unwind.

Alcohol is a very versatile substance but it does take a toll on our ability to perform each day. Our fitness at all levels can be affected. Your diary will highlight the drinking you enjoy most and the drinking that is simply habitual. Knowing this information you can make a decision on when you would like to drink most in the future and your incentive to act on this decision will be the knowledge that you will feel better and you will perform better in the future.

There is no need to think that you must drastically restrict your alcohol intake or feel that you are depriving yourself. The object of this exercise is to analyse the 'quality' of your drinking. Drink when you enjoy it and when alcohol is performing the function you want it to – you are being sociable or relaxing – and then really enjoy it. But recognize when this moment has passed and you are drinking out of habit because habitual drinking usually undermines good work done elsewhere.

Energy levels

Alcohol can make you feel energetic but because of the sugar it contains it will cause a rise and then a fall in your blood sugar levels leading to fatigue. The drop in blood sugar explains why you feel hungry towards the end of a night of drinking or why you feel so low on energy the morning after. Drinking less or drinking more slowly makes it easier to be aware of and to manage your energy levels more carefully.

Alcohol, hangovers and your fitness programme

The final word on alcohol considers how your drinking habits are impacting on your exercise progress. Again, your diaries will highlight clear connections between nights out on the tiles and your ability to follow your exercise programme. One important question to consider in relation to your short- and long-term progress is, should you exercise with a hangover?

We have all been there. You have had a really good week and all you need to do to put the icing on the cake is to complete your workout on Sunday morning and you will feel great about yourself. But the lure of a Saturday night out is just too much. you have worked hard and you deserve to let your hair down so you throw caution to the wind and just relax into your evening out. One thing leads to another and you wake up on Sunday feeling like exercise is the last thing on your mind. So what should you do? Roll over, curl up and hope you feel better later? Or bite the bullet, get out there and face the day?

Hangovers, like the drinks that cause them, come in many varieties and degrees of seriousness. One thing you can be sure of is that after a night on the booze, physically, you will be dehydrated and your blood sugar/energy levels will be at rock bottom. Alcohol contains ethanol which is a diuretic and causes you to lose a lot of fluid – more fluid than you drink – so no matter how much water you manage to get into your body between drinks, you are bound to be at least a little dehydrated first thing the next morning. The feeling of dehydration will contribute to your lethargy, your dry mouth and the banging in your head.

Alcohol also contains a lot of sugar which will initially cause the blood sugar to rise. Drinking in excess causes this rise to be too great for the body to function effectively so it will produce insulin to lower the amount of sugar in the blood. The net effect, particularly after a night's sleep, is that blood sugar is low. Alcohol also lacks any nutrients beneficial to the body and actually robs the body of some of the vitamins and minerals it needs to carry out its daily functions. You particularly lose a lot of potassium and sodium with your increased trips to the toilet. These chemicals are essential for optimum function of nerves and muscles and will be at their lowest levels following a night on the tiles leading to nausea, fatigue and headaches. So all in all, it is not surprising that you do not feel on tip top form!

Enough of the bad news. The good news is that, if you are careful, taking some exercise can get you back to feeling normal quicker then if you lounge around feeling sorry for yourself.

Shake off your hangover and feel fighting fit fast

First things first, if you feel sick, take something to settle your stomach. Although not normally recommended, fizzy drinks are an effective solution here as the bubbles calm your tummy and the sweetness will raise your blood sugar and give you some energy. The caffeine in many fizzy drinks will act as a diuretic so make sure you drink some water as soon as you can to begin the process of rehydrating. If your stomach feels fragile but you feel safe to eat, some fruit will kick-start your metabolism.

If your symptoms are less serious in your stomach but you have a thick head, drink plenty of water and eat something slightly more substantial. Eggs and toast are a popular hangover choice as the toast provides carbohydrates for energy and the eggs contain cysteine which helps to mop up free radicals. Free radicals are cells in the body that can cause damage but are usually dealt with by the liver. If the liver is not functioning well, as might be the case thanks to excessive alcohol, you may have more free radicals in your system than is good for you and the eggs will help to rectify this situation.

Once you have stabilized your nausea, given your body some energy and hydrated your shrivelled cells, you can think about getting your body moving. It may still not be top of your agenda, but exercise will make you breathe which will increase the oxygen and blood flow around your body. This will increase the speed at which toxins are broken down and eliminated and so will get you feeling better quickly. Exercise also boosts your body's production of mood improving endorphins which can be drastically depleted by excessive alcohol, one of the reasons why you can feel a bit out of sorts after a big night out.

When you feel hungover, set your exercise goals low. To think about completing your normal routine will only make you feel tired and will put you off doing anything. Plan to do just a little bit and then see how you get on. Chances are, once you are out doing something, you will be capable of more than you imagined. It is getting yourself going that is important here. Put your usual kit on to show yourself that you are serious and to tell your brain that you are moving on from hangover mode to exercise mode and that by the time you finish you will feel better in the same way you always feel good after you exercise.

Take some water with you and begin with a gentle walk. Choose a route with open space and clean air and breathe deeply to get plenty of oxygen in to help clear the toxins out. Stretch gently as you walk to lengthen muscles and improve your posture. Begin running by picking a spot to run to and then resting and walking when you get there. This low intensity interval training will encourage the heart, lungs and muscles to become accustomed to working a bit harder and will give you a chance to monitor how you are feeling without overdoing it. Providing you feel OK, you can gradually increase the distances that you run and, if you are feeling really good, carry on with as much of your programme as you feel comfortable with.

One word of caution. Although it is generally safe to exercise on a hangover and it will help you to feel better, you might not feel fully fighting fit after a night out so aim to use your workout to maintain fitness rather than to push yourself and develop new fitness levels. Treat the workout as part of your overall hangover cure, which includes eating and drinking sensibly, resting and looking after yourself for the day.

Exercise on a hangover: when to go and when to say no

If your hangover is light and you just feel a bit 'fuzzy' you are safe to exercise though you should pay a little more attention than normal to hydration levels and energy levels. Drink water steadily until you are going to the toilet regularly and producing pale urine. Eat something that will sustain you during your workout and refuel as soon as you can on your return. Around 20–30 minutes of moderate exercise should be just right to get you feeling human again.

If your hangover is moderate and you have the obligatory headache, dry mouth, feelings of sickness and lethargy, exercise could be just the thing to see off all your symptoms. Your senses may be a little dulled so it is a good idea to follow a familiar routine rather than having to deal with anything new when you are not at your most responsive. Begin gently and regularly review how you are feeling. Aim for 10–15 minutes of gentle exercise to begin with and if you feel worse at any stage, lower the intensity or stop completely.

When it comes to exercising on a hangover, be sensible. If you can barely stand and everything is blurry, it is not the morning for a workout. Focus on rehydrating, re-energising and rest. Schedule a walk for mid-afternoon when you are a bit more stable and the fresh air and movement will see off the last of your symptoms.

Using your diaries to shape the future

So, now that you know the value of keeping diaries and recognize what to look out for, start collecting the information on what is going on with you, your fitness, your exercise, your food and your body. There are templates for the diaries at the back of the book, or you may find it easier to format your own. You can use separate notebooks for keeping diaries, just make sure that you write down everything so it can be analysed, reviewed and modified where necessary.

Step 1

Establish your current behaviour around fitness and food, and the results that go with this behaviour, namely your current body shape, energy levels and personal happiness.

Step 2

Begin making gradual changes to your current behaviour, based on what you want to achieve and what will fit into your life. Chapters 7 and 8 give you plenty of exercise and food options which will enable you to try out some new ideas and experiment with different approaches until you find the one that works for you.

Step 3

Continually monitor and review what you do and the results you get. Keep experimenting around what works best for you as you never know just how good you could look and feel unless you test a number of approaches.

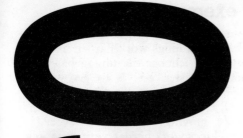

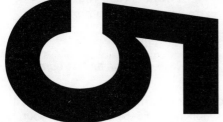

05

the exercises

In this chapter you will learn:
- to recognize different types of exercise
- to understand what each exercise will do for you
- how to perform each exercise.

Cardiovascular exercise

Cardiovascular (CV) means heart and lungs. CV exercise is anything that makes the heart and lungs work harder. You can choose the intensity and you can choose the timing based on what you want to achieve, but step one is to get started. Walking, running, skipping, swimming, cycling, rowing, stepping and dancing are all CV exercises and there are many more. You get your body moving beyond the everyday requirements, your heart and lungs work harder, your metabolic rate rises, your muscles use extra energy and you burn fat.

Fitness Myth 1

Low intensity CV exercise is best as it keeps me in the 'fat-burning zone'.

The 'fat-burning zone' as described on many pieces of fitness equipment usually suggests working at 55–65 per cent of your maximum heart rate (the highest number of heart beats per minute that you can achieve when you are working to your full effort level). The reasoning is that when working between 55–65 per cent of your maximum heart rate the body is working with a balance of energy between fat and muscle energy that is optimum for burning fat. This is good, however, the fat-burning zone is not the only zone where you will burn fat, you simply burn it in different proportions as you exercise to different intensity. If you work harder than 65 per cent of your maximum heart rate, you will burn more fat calories overall. In short, for maximum fat loss, work harder.

Let's face it, it makes sense doesn't it? Can you really expect to lose more weight by working less hard and keeping your effort level below 65 per cent of what it could be? If you have any doubts at all in this area, use your diary and conduct a controlled experiment. Try exercising in the fat-burning zone for six-to-eight weeks and monitor the results. Then exercise for six-to-eight weeks working as hard as you can during every CV workout and monitor the results of this activity. By comparing the two ways of working, you will be able to see which works best and how you wish to proceed from here.

Strength training

Strength training means putting your muscles under an extra load beyond that which they are used to in order to tone you up and make you stronger. Strength training does not mean lifting huge weights and bulking up. The weights that you train with and the pattern of sets and repetitions that you do can be adjusted to bring you the specific results you are looking for when shaping your body, so do not be afraid of strength training. Once again your diary can be invaluable as it will show you the results of the changes you make. If you are not achieving your desired results, modify your pattern of exercise and monitor it until you get precisely what you want.

Fitness Myth 2

Training with weights will make me bulky.

To achieve muscle bulk you need very heavy weights and a training regime of short sets where you can only perform a few repetitions of each exercise before having to rest and recover. If you work with moderate weights that allow you to perform between 15 and 20 repetitions with good technique before you have to rest, you will strengthen, shape and tone your muscles without becoming bulky.

Flexibility training

Flexibility training is probably the most commonly overlooked part of any fitness programme, possibly because the benefits of stretching are not felt as obviously as the benefits of CV or strength training. With CV training you can get quite tired, you breathe hard, you sweat and you can sense the calories burning – you really feel that you are doing something positive for your health. With strength training it feels good to flex your muscles and move the weights to tone different areas, and the glow of a well-worked body part reassures you that you are making good progress with your fitness. Stretching is often viewed differently. It is seen as the area of fitness that you should pay attention to because you read somewhere that it was important to keep yourself supple. But maybe it doesn't feel like it is doing much, it does not give you that instant buzz like other parts of your routine do, so gradually it slips off the exercise radar.

For flexibility training to become an integral part of your programme, it has to be given some context in your overall fitness plan and lifestyle. Otherwise, you just will not do it. So let's think about why you might want to do it and how you can fit it in if you do want to do it.

Most exercises involve contracting muscles to create movement. If you repeatedly contract muscle groups without ever stretching these areas you can negatively affect the balance of your body and the way you look. Exaggerated examples of these effects can clearly be seen with some body builders. If they spend a disproportionate amount of time working on the parts of their body they can see in the mirror as they exercise, primarily their chest, shoulders and arms, these areas are frequently contracted under a heavy load. Without the proper balance of working the rest of the body and particularly without regular stretching of the muscle groups they are focusing on, the muscles can become shortened over time. Because the areas worked, the 'mirror muscles' in this case, are all towards the front of the body, this progressive shortening can lead to the body being pulled forwards into a stoop that can look ape like in its extreme, and can potentially lead to long-term injury.

It is very unlikely that you will be taking things to this extreme level but the example illustrates the point that you need to balance muscle contractions with some stretching.

The way we live our modern lives puts a lot of stress on various parts of our bodies. We sit down for a large proportion of the time which can lead to shortening of the muscles at the backs of our legs. We spend a lot of time hunched over our computers or sitting in our cars, which can lead to a variety of neck, shoulder and back problems. The many hours that we spent distractedly chatting on the phone can mean hours of sitting or standing in a compromised position which can, over time, take its toll.

The easiest way to fit stretching into the schedule is simply to stretch muscles immediately after you have used them. If you do some cycling, stretch out your legs and back when you have finished. If you do some press-ups, stretch out your chest and arms. You need a moment to recover from each exercise before you move on to the next one so why not use this time usefully and stretch along the way? By working and then stretching each area of the body, you maintain the overall balance of your body which helps you to stand upright, look taller, appear thinner, breathe more easily and generally look healthier.

Regular stretching gives you the chance to realign everything in your body and to undo the damage caused by everyday life. One regular weekly stretching session for your whole body will straighten you out and remind your limbs of where they should be to keep you safe and injury free, and keep you supple as you go about your daily business. Added to this, a few neck stretches, shoulder rolls, chest and leg stretches performed throughout the day will keep the negative side-effects of modern working life at bay.

Two good reasons to stretch:

- Long lean muscles lead to lithe looks.
- Stretching can balance the ravages, tension and stress of modern life.

Use the notes you make in your exercise diary to determine what stretches will benefit you most, and how you can best fit them into your routine. Examine the exercises you are doing and the results you are getting and consider what stretches could be necessary to balance and enhance these results.

Core training

Core training focuses on the muscles deep inside the abdominal area. These muscles are designed to stabilize the pelvis and help keep correct body alignment for safe and injury-free movement. In the past, exercise routines tended to focus on everything but this area. It was fine to exercise your arms, legs, shoulders, back and aim for the perfect six-pack but less attention was paid to how these exercises were performed. The result was injury in many cases. On investigation, it was found that exercising your body without paying attention to the core area was like building a house without putting in proper foundations. It looks good from the outside, but is it safe and built to last? Your core area is like the foundations of your body. If you pay attention to this part of your training, everything else is safer and more effective. Controlling your stomach muscles at a deep level will give you good posture and correct body alignment. This enables you to perform all your exercises with the minimal risk of injury and the maximum chance of positive results over time.

The beauty of this part of your exercise routine is that you can do it wherever and whenever you want. By sitting or standing up straight and tightening your pelvic floor, you can activate your deep stomach muscles. you will notice that your posture instantly improves. You sit taller and straighter and your shoulders move back and down to a more relaxed position. Practise this frequently as the more often you put yourself in this position, the better the ability of these muscles to hold you there for longer will be. They are endurance muscles, they need to be gradually persuaded to work over longer periods of time. The more you make them work, the more they will work for you.

Stability and balance training, functional training and sport-specific training

The classifications of these types of training are slightly more specialized and so you need to consider when and if you include these elements as part of your individual routine.

Stability and balance training, making use of kit such as fitballs, medicine balls, wobble boards and instability discs, is designed to increase the efficiency of the signals transmitted from your brain to various muscles in order that you can use or recruit muscles more quickly, recruit more muscles in a particular area or recruit these muscles for longer.

Functional training and sport-specific training involve fitness routines tailored very specifically to certain ends. Functional fitness is training for everyday activities – to make what you do every day easier and safer. Sport-specific training means tailoring your workout for your particular event. If you have weak ankles, for example, walking over rough terrain is functional training as it will exercise the major and minor muscles in and around the ankle area. If you play netball you may incorporate exercises such as press-ups with a hand clap to increase passing power, or short directional sprints to improve your agility around the court. These elements of an exercise programme may not be for everyone but by monitoring your routine and its results with your diary, you will be able to clearly see if they will benefit you.

Rest and recovery

This is the part of your fitness routine you can really look forward to. If you are training regularly and effectively, you need to factor in time to recover. During your workouts you place demands on your body beyond the normal run of the daily routine. You encourage your heart to beat faster, your lungs to work harder and your muscles to take on loads they're not used to. This is called overload and we do it because, by overloading, you encourage your body to make changes and become stronger. Your body is clever and likes to be efficient so if it has found something hard work, it will endeavour to change and adapt in order that, if it were to find itself in the same situation in the future, it would not find things so tough.

This is the reason why you need to keep moving your goals forwards if you want to continue your progress. After a while, your body will have made sufficient changes to be able to cope with your initial challenges quite easily so if you want further progress, you need a new challenge, you need more overload. Alternatively, if you are happy with your results at this point you can continue to use the same programme to maintain these results.

The body's adaptation, growth and development for the long-term takes place following your workout, not during it, so you must allow the body time to make these changes by taking rest or recovery days. This is why exercising every other day is effective. You overload your body during your workout on day one and stimulate the changes that take place on day two. You then exercise again on day three when your body has had a chance to become stronger and more efficient, then recover from this and make further adaptations on day four. And so on.

You can recover from most workouts with a single day's rest. If you have had a particularly tough exercise session, you may need a couple of days to recover and get the best out of your next session. Use your judgement here. If you feel you have not properly recovered from a workout, give it another day or you will risk encountering the law of diminishing returns where you may train more, but because your body has not fully recovered from a previous workout, you do not get the results you otherwise may see. Worse than this, if you are not fully recovered, you could injure yourself.

If you look at your schedule at the beginning of the week and discover that the only days you have for exercising are consecutive days, structure these workouts to contain different activities on each day. You could run on the first day and cycle on the next. Or swim on day one and use the trampoline on day two. With your strength training a general rule of thumb for exercise on consecutive days is to work the upper body one day and the lower body the next. Or focus on different muscle groups on different days. A guideline here is to perform exercises where you are pushing resistance away from your body on day one – shoulder press, tricep extensions, press-ups – and use exercises that involve pulling resistance towards your body on day two – pull ups, rows or bicep curls. The next section will explain exactly which exercises target different areas of your body to help you plan each and every workout for maximum effectiveness.

> Rest days are also crucial for your state of mind. You need to be focused on your exercise programme but you need to live your life as well. If you plan carefully when you will exercise, and when you will not, you will make your workouts effective and then enjoy your rest days and use them for doing something completely different.

CV training – the exercises

Walking

Why do it?

Walking is a great way to get started with your fitness programme. You can easily fit extra walking into your daily routine and create a tough workout in a short space of time.

How do I do it?

Walk with good posture keeping your shoulders relaxed and with your top half in an upright position. Clench your bottom muscles for good position and to get maximum toning benefits in this area. Swing your arms for a vigorous workout and breathe deeply as you go. Walk with purpose and set yourself time and distance targets to keep you motivated. If you walk as part of your daily routine, aim to get from A to B as fast as you can, whenever you can. If you walk as part of a more formal fitness routine, begin by setting a benchmark by choosing a set distance and seeing how long it takes you to cover. Alternatively, if you're using a treadmill, set a target time and see how far you can go in that time.

Progressions

For maximum fitness progress, aim to walk further or faster with every workout. When you are comfortable with your progress walking on the flat, vary the terrain by walking in areas that are hilly or by using the incline facility on a treadmill. The steeper the climb, the tougher your workout will be.

Skipping

Why do it?

Skipping is a great exercise for raising the heart rate quickly and provides a good workout for the heart and lungs. It is also a completely portable workout allowing you to burn some calories wherever and whenever you want to.

How do I do it?

A plastic or leather rope will help you build up the best momentum and you must make sure you buy one that is the right size for you. If the rope is too long or too short you will not be able to find a comfortable rhythm. Make sure that you have sufficient space around you, and above you before you begin. Stand on one foot with the rope behind you. Bring the rope around over your head and jump off of one leg, over the rope and onto the other leg. Bring the rope round again and jump over it onto the starting leg. Repeat this and try to improve on the number of skips you can do every time you try.

Progressions

Skipping can be as hard as you want to make it. To make it easier you can skip with two feet together and add a small jump between rotations of the rope. To increase the intensity of your workout you can simply speed up your rate of skipping and aim for as many skips as you can in one minute or two minutes with short rests between your efforts. If you are feeling energetic and brave you can even try to skip with two feet together and rotate the rope twice round for every jump that you make.

Step-ups

If you are short of time or lacking in motivation to go outside in the cold weather, this is the perfect exercise solution. All you need is one or two steps or stairs and you can give yourself a really good cardiovascular workout which will help to tone up your legs and your bottom.

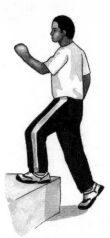

figure 3 step-ups

Option 1 – Low intensity maintaining fitness

Find a step that is about the same size as a household staircase and simply step up with the left foot, up with the right, down with the left and down with the right keeping a comfortable and regular rhythm. Change the leading leg after 30 seconds and rest after 2 minutes of stepping.

Option 2 – Moderate intensity for quicker results

Follow the same pattern as above but use a slightly larger step, increase your speed slightly and only swap the leading leg after one minute. Keep the top half of your body upright by working your stomach muscles. Your shoulders should be back and relaxed and your chest should not be flopping down towards your thighs.

Option 3 – Higher intensity for fastest gains

Either find a larger step, a bench, or step up two stairs at a time. Even though the step is now bigger, do not be tempted to push your arms off your thighs to help you up. It is the lower body that should be working hardest complemented by a strong swinging action of the arms which will help you keep your rhythm. Step up and down briskly for a minute and then change the leading leg. Rest for 30 seconds between each 2 minutes of stepping and complete four sets for each leg.

Running

Why do it?

The original and, in many people's opinion, the best way to exercise effectively for fast results. It is totally portable and you do not require any equipment, just some comfortable clothing and the correct footwear. And even the footwear is optional under certain circumstances; there is no better workout for getting back to nature with your fitness than running barefoot along the beach. Running involves the whole body so is a very efficient way to exercise and by planning the duration and intensity of your workouts, you can design your results in advance.

How do I do it?

Running is accessible to practically everyone but there are still a few things to look out for to make your workouts the most effective they can be and to keep you safe and injury free. Focus on your posture and begin running with your body upright, eyes forwards and your shoulders back and relaxed. If it helps, you may want to walk a few strides with good posture and then gradually break into a run keeping your good position. Use your arms by driving your elbows back to help propel you forwards and lift the knees on every step. Breathe deeply to get plenty of oxygen to the working muscles. If your aim is to shift a lot of weight, running can be quite demanding on your joints so it is always a good idea to begin with a lower impact exercise like cycling and then trampolining in order to strengthen muscles and connective tissue and to increase stability at joints before progressing to full impact running. When you do run, begin with very short bursts of running mixed with walking to recover until you feel confident to gradually increase the amount of time you spend running.

How long should I run for?

The beauty of running is that you can do it whenever you fancy. If you have plenty of time you can go for a long slow run to work on your long distance endurance. These long runs are great for fitness and also brilliant for taking in some scenery, stimulating your imagination and letting your mind wander. When you have less time you can go for a shorter, faster run to really get your heart and lungs working. If you spend these shorter workouts on sprint training, hill training or interval training you can give yourself as tough a workout in 10 or 15 minutes as you can with an hour-long slower run.

Cycling

Why do it?

Cycling uses the large muscles of the lower body to work your heart and lungs and if you gauge the intensity of your workout correctly you can achieve quick fitness gains and burn body fat efficiently.

How do I get started?

Outdoor cycling is a great way to get around and incorporate some functional fitness into your weekly routine. Providing you are safe and confident, you can cycle to work, to the shops, or to see friends. Before you go anywhere, check your bike is roadworthy. If you are unsure what to look for, take it to a cycle shop and ask them to service it for you. Ensure that you have a crash helmet, and that you use it, and also that you wear suitable clothes for cycling with nothing hanging loose that could get caught anywhere. If you need to carry anything as you cycle either have a basket fitted or use a backpack rather than dangling anything over the handlebars.

Plan your routes carefully based on what you are trying to achieve. If you are cycling to work you will probably want to go the most direct route or the quietest route. If you are cycling to meet friends you may want to take a diverted route in order to get a bit more of a workout. If you are out for a ride purely to work on your fitness you may want to plan in some quiet or straight sections where you can cycle faster for more of a workout, or even take a hilly route to challenge your legs and your lungs.

When you are cycling pay attention to your posture and sit up straight rather than slouching over the handlebars. An upright position will enable you to get more muscles involved in the action, primarily the large muscles of your bottom, and will also protect your lower back and keep your lungs open, allowing you to breathe more easily. Pedal evenly with both legs and to make you work a bit harder, try to stay in the saddle as much as possible. Keep your shoulders and your arms relaxed and always have some water with you. If possible, have a phone with you, just in case.

Isn't it scary out there on the busy roads?

The roads can be busy but if you like to cycle you can plan around this issue to find quiet routes or quiet times to go for your ride. If the idea of the traffic really puts you off you can cycle in the gym and use the programmes on the machine to simulate the changing conditions of an outdoor bike ride.

Trampolining

Why do it?

Using a small trampoline or rebounder is a great way to burn some calories by working your whole body but without putting your joints under the same stresses as they are subject to when running. The trampoline cushions the impact, making it a good option for anyone with any problems with their ankles, knees or hips.

What is a good workout on the trampoline?

Start by marching on the trampoline and gradually raising your knees higher and higher at the front. When you feel warmed up, slowly lower the height to which you lift your knees and then begin to jog gently. Bring your arms into the movement and increase the speed of the running to make your workout more challenging. Short bursts of 'sprinting' will really make your heart and lungs work hard. An alternative way to work on the trampoline is to begin with small jumps keeping your legs together and using your ankles to lift you into the air. Gradually bend your knees more and more to make the jumps bigger and swing your arms to achieve the biggest and most energetic jumps.

To keep your workouts interesting, use a variety of techniques on the trampoline and vary the intensity by doing timed bursts of low, moderate and high intensity work with short recovery periods of gentle bouncing in between.

What else can I do with this trampoline?

Standing on the trampoline provides you with an unstable base which you can use when performing some of your strength training exercises. If you would like to do some extra work on your core stability muscles and balance, stand on your trampoline while you do exercises such as the shoulder press, tricep extensions, bicep curls, shoulder raises or squats.

Stair runs

Why do it?

Another portable solution for a good workout. You can use stairs at home, at work, around town or on escalators to sneak some exercise into your weekly routine.

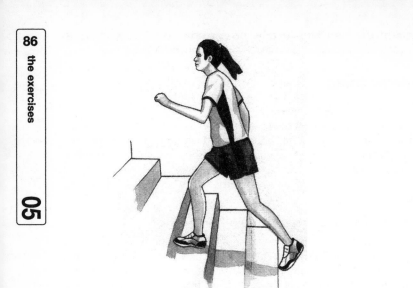

figure 4 stair runs

Will running up stairs really make a difference?

Anything that gets your heart and lungs working will make a difference. If you walk up stairs as part of your regular commute or working pattern, running up the same stairs will burn some extra calories. You can also devise a specific stair run workout which you can do at home or on some local steps, providing it is safe to do so.

When you run up stairs, ensure your posture is good. Your body should be upright and your shoulders relaxed. Lift your knees as you go up the stairs and keep on the balls of your feet. Swing your arms to help with the rhythm of your movement. To begin with, jog up a flight of 10 to 20 steps and walk back down to the bottom as recovery. To make the workout more difficult, use the same flight of stairs and run up them two at a time. Running quickly up single steps will give you a really good CV workout. Running the stairs two at a time will still work your heart and lungs and the bigger strides will give you an added toning workout for the lower body muscles – bottom, thighs and calves.

Any special advice for this one?

Obviously there are some inherent dangers involved with stairs so take care to plant your feet carefully on every step that you take as you run up, and walk down gently as you recover. If there is a banister, use it if you feel you need to and take a rest if you feel at all wobbly.

Rowing

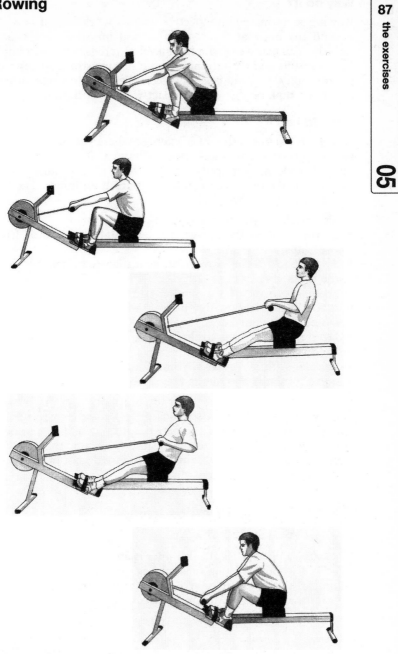

figure 5 rowing

Why do it?

Rowing is an incredibly effective way to work lots of muscles around the body at the same time and improve your fitness quickly. You can work to a high level of intensity for incredible fitness results and fat burning without putting strain on any part of your body. You will be supported either by a rowing machine or a boat, making this a low impact way to work out.

How do I do it?

Rowing is the one form of CV exercise where you are advised to ask a professional to check your technique. If you are slightly out of position, you could hamper your fitness gains, create muscle imbalances over time or do yourself an injury. The key points to look out for are:

- Sit upright as you row.
- At the front of the movement, lean slightly forwards from your hips.
- At the back of the movement, lean slightly backwards from the hips.
- From the front of the stroke, drive through the legs and follow this quickly with a pull of the arms.
- Do not lock your knees.
- From the back of the stroke, straighten your arms before you bend your legs.
- Breathe with a regular rhythm, ideally breathing in as you move forwards and out as you drive backwards.

Once you feel comfortable with the technique you can mix up your workout with timed sessions of faster and slower rowing with short recovery periods in between. It is a good idea to have your technique checked regularly just to ensure that, as you increase the intensity of your workouts, you do not move out of position.

Elliptical trainer or cross trainer

Why do it?

The cross trainer or elliptical trainer is an effective way to burn calories without stressing or straining any joints. The machine supports the weight of your body leaving you free to concentrate on how hard you are working.

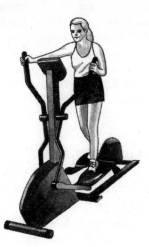

figure 6 the cross trainer

How do I do it?

Using the elliptical trainer is very simple. Keep good posture and breathe regularly for an efficient workout with great results. Each machine has programmed settings to add variety and intensity. Stride forwards to work the front of your thighs and backwards if you are looking to work the backs of your thighs a little more. Squeeze your bottom at all times to tone this area and to give you a good position.

Swimming

Why do it?

The buoyancy of the water supports your bodyweight so almost anyone can swim without pain and there are a variety of strokes to choose from allowing you to alter the intensity of your workouts and avoid boredom.

How do I do it?

Swimming is another exercise where professional advice will stand you in good stead and enable you to get the best fitness results possible. Even if you are relatively new to swimming you can achieve effective results by challenging yourself to swim faster than you are used to for a few lengths and then allowing yourself a couple of lengths to recover.

Treat swimming as you would any other form of exercise. You may be working out in the water but you still need to drink to keep yourself hydrated. You also need to stretch at the end of your swimming session so allow yourself time to dry off and stretch out before you get changed.

Alternate leg squat thrusts

A variation on the old 'Superstars' favourite, this exercise is good for training the heart and lungs with the added bonus of working the upper body and core stability muscles.

Take up a position with your hands and feet on the floor as if you were about to begin a set of press-ups. Make sure your stomach muscles are switched on and your body is in a straight line from your shoulders to your ankles. Extend your neck in front of you so that your head is in line with your body, and lower your chest so that your shoulder blades are retracted – you should not feel rounded at the shoulders. Bend your left knee and bring your left foot up so that it is on the floor underneath your hip. This is your starting position. The exercise is to move both legs at the same time so that you end up with the left leg straight and the right leg bent with your right foot beneath you. Be careful that you do not sag at the middle as you progress through the set – your stomach should work hard throughout to prevent your back arching at any stage.

Aim to do about 40 repetitions and then break before repeating. You should move with quite a quick and regular rhythm for the duration of each set.

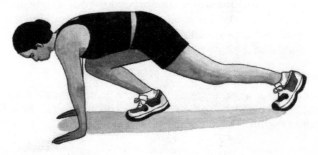

figure 7 alternate leg squat thrusts

Strength training – lower body exercises

Please note that for all strength training exercises, where dumbbells are mentioned, any resistance will do. Many of the exercises can be performed with a resistance band or with bottles of water or even tins of beans for resistance. The only stipulation is that you use resistance that challenges you for maximum results.

Squats

Why do it?

With this single exercise you can develop the whole of the lower body as well as working on your core strength and lumbar stability.

What do I need to do?

Grab a weight in each hand – dumbbells, water bottles or heavy bags will do – and stand up straight with your feet shoulder-width apart and shoulders back and relaxed. Your neck should be in line with your spine and your eyes forward and slightly down. Tighten up around the stomach area and then bend at the hips and knees to lower into the squat position. Make sure that when you perform the exercise your knees do not travel forwards beyond the line of your toes. Lower your bottom until your thighs are almost parallel with the floor and do not let your shoulders drop too far forwards. Now stand upright again without locking out at the knees. Keep your stomach muscles tight and your shoulders back with your head in line with your body at all times.

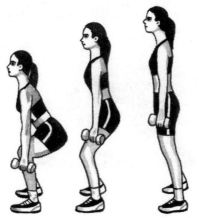

figure 8 the squat

Anything to look out for with this one?

Some people feel pressure on their knees during this exercise. If this happens simply widen your stance and turn your toes outwards before you begin. Wide-leg squats can be slightly easier on the knees.

Wide-leg squats

Also known as ballet squats or plie squats, these are very good for toning the bottom and thighs.

Grab a dumbbell in each hand and take up a wide stance with your feet well apart and your toes turned outwards to an angle of 45 degrees each. Hold the dumbbells in front of you and stand upright with your shoulders back and down and your stomach working to keep your back in its neutral position. Now bend at the hips so that your bottom travels behind you a little and then bend the knees to move into the squat position. Ensure that your knees travel towards your toes – and not towards each other into a 'knock-kneed' position – and that they stay behind the line of your toes. Your stomach should work throughout to ensure that your top half remains upright and the weights do not pull you forwards causing you to round your shoulders. Keep the exercise slow, pause at the bottom of the movement briefly and then stand upright without locking out your knees. Repeat 15 times and then rest before attempting set two.

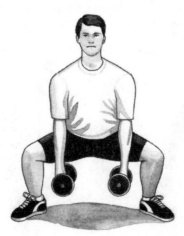

figure 9 the wide leg squat

You will know the exercise is correct if you can feel you are working your inner thighs and the backs of your legs. If you do not feel this you need to sit into the exercise further rather than allowing your weight to move forward.

Lunges

Why do it?

A great exercise for strengthening the lower body and improving balance. The basic exercise uses lots of muscles in the lower body as well as stability muscles around the body, making it a good exercise for toning and generating muscle tissue to raise your metabolism, as well as a good exercise to improve your posture.

How do I do it?

Stand with feet hip-width apart and take a large step forward with one foot. Keep your body upright and your weight evenly distributed between your legs. Raise your back heel and stand still here for a moment. This is your start/finish position. Bend both legs so that the back knee travels towards the ground. Make sure that you bend the back leg enough to allow the front knee to stay behind the front toe. At the bottom of the movement you should have a 90-degree angle at both knees and

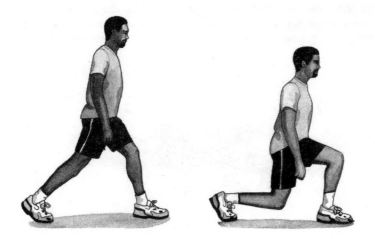

figure 10 the lunge

your hips, with your torso upright. Straighten up the legs without locking out the knees and repeat 15–20 times on each leg before swapping the legs around.

How do I progress it?

Lunges can be performed with a dumbbell or weight in each hand to make your legs and your stability muscles work harder.

Side leg lifts

An exercise to isolate and target the sides of the thighs and the bottom.

Lie on the floor on your side ensuring that your hips are vertically aligned. The arm that is nearest the floor should be extended underneath your head with your head resting on it. Your neck must be in line with your body to prevent any pulling on the spine. Place the hand of your upper arm in front of your stomach for balance. Now move the top hip forward slightly so that your hips are at a 75-degree angle to the floor. With this angle at the hips you will be sure that as you raise your top leg towards the ceiling you will be working into the bottom rather than the front of the hip. The final check to ensure you work the desired area is to keep your foot flat and parallel with the ground as you raise your leg. Do not point your toes upwards at any stage. Lift the leg slowly in a straight line without letting it come in front of your body. Pause at the top of the movement and squeeze the muscles to get the most out of the exercise before slowly lowering the leg. Repeat 15 times and then swap legs.

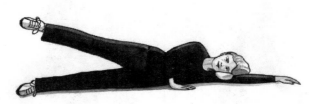

figure 11 the side leg lift

To make the exercise more difficult you can loop a resistance band around your ankles. The range of movement will be slightly less but the effort level will be greater.

Squat jumps

Why do it?

Helps to improve dynamic strength in the lower body, improves balance and works the heart and lungs. It is a great portable workout requiring minimal room, just a bit of space above you. And it is a tough one!

How do I do it?

Stand up straight with your feet shoulder-width apart and your toes pointing forwards. Bend at the knees and lower your bottom as if you were about to sit down, making sure that you keep your weight on your heels and that your knees do not travel forwards beyond the line of your toes. Lower yourself until you have a 90-degree angle at your knees and then, using your arms to gain momentum, spring up as high as you can, pointing your toes to give you maximum height. Land with two feet together, make sure you are balanced and then repeat the sequence without pausing. You should aim for 20 consecutive jumps at a rate of one jump every two seconds. Make sure that you hold your stomach in tight throughout as this will help to prevent over-balancing.

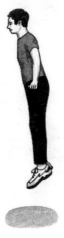
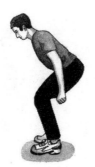

figure 12 the squat jump

Lunge jumps

Why do it?

A really great workout for cardiovascular fitness which also tones up the legs and the bottom.

How do I do it?

Stand with your feet hip-width apart and take a big step forward with one foot. Now bend both legs so the front knee travels forward – but only as far as the line of the front toe – and the back knee travels towards the floor (careful not to bang your knee on the floor). Tighten your stomach muscles to help you balance and keep your top half upright – do not lean your chest forwards at any point during the exercise. At the lowest point of the movement you should have 90-degree angles at both knees and at your hips. Once you feel you are balanced, spring up through both legs, change your leading leg whilst you are in mid-air and land with the opposite leg forwards. Your feet should still be hip-distance apart and you should be able to land with balance and lower yourself gently into the lunge position. Repeat this 20 times, changing legs each time you jump.

This one is a bit tough – is it necessary?

Lunge jumps can be used as a toning exercise that gives fast results. It is also an exercise which will make you work hard to balance and improve the alignment of your body. It will also improve dynamic strength in the lower body for sprinting and

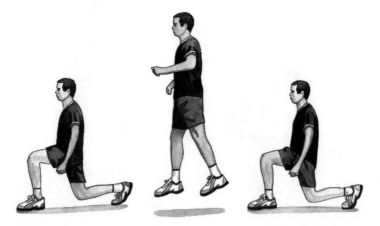

figure 13 the lunge jump

jumping sports. Once you have mastered the technique you can make it more difficult by holding progressively larger dumbbells in each hand as you perform the jumps but be careful not to overbalance. If you want a challenging exercise with fast results, this is one for you.

Single leg squat

Why do it?

A great strength exercise for runners, cyclists, jumpers and others who need good balance and strong, shapely legs.

How do I do it?

Make sure you have plenty of space around you and then stand on one leg with your other leg just behind you with the toe gently in contact with the ground. You can hold your arms out to the sides to help with your balance. Tighten up at the stomach and then, keeping your hips level by tightening your bottom muscles, bend your supporting leg to around 90 degrees without letting the knee travel forwards beyond the line of your toe. To do this you need to bend at the hips and allow your bottom to travel backwards and down. This keeps the angle at the knee shallow and will avoid putting a lot of stress on this joint. As you bend your knees, your upper body should remain

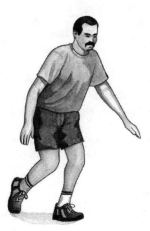

figure 14 the single leg squat

relatively upright rather than pitching too far forward and you must engage your core stability muscles strongly to ensure this is the case. When you have reached the bottom of the movement, slowly stand up on one leg, controlling the movement with your stomach and leg. Complete 10 squats on one leg and then swap.

Strength training – upper body exercises

Press-up

Why do it?

The press-up is a simple way of exercising a lot of muscles, particularly in the upper body, in one movement. You can work your chest, shoulders, arms and stomach together, making it a very time-efficient exercise to have in your routine. It is also one of the most portable strength exercises around.

How do I do it?

Press-ups on the ground are difficult for a beginner to do correctly so use a bench or table to raise your hands higher than your feet and make the exercise a little easier. Place your hands on the bench about shoulder-width apart. Move your feet away from the bench until your body is straight from shoulders to ankles with your shoulders over your hands. You should feel that you are holding your stomach muscles tight so that you do not sag in the middle. Drop your chest a little so that you can feel a slight tension between your shoulder blades and lengthen your neck so that your head is in line with your body and not sagging down looking towards your feet. Now bend your arms and lower your chest towards the bench, and straighten them to return to the starting position without losing the straight line of your body. Make sure that you do not round your shoulders as you push up from the bench or lock out your elbows at the top of the movement.

What are the benefits?

An effective exercise for strengthening and toning and, when done correctly, the press up will help improve posture over time.

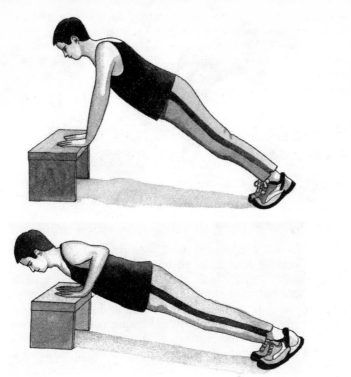

figure 15 the press-up

Single arm row

Why do it?

To strengthen the major muscles of the back and arms to ensure good posture and a strong body. Working these big muscles is a great way to get your metabolism firing and burning calories.

How do I do it?

Stand in front of a bench or table with a dumbbell or other weight in one hand and the other hand on the bench so that your weight is distributed between two legs and one arm. Ensure that you are bent over at the hips and not the waist so that your lower back is in a neutral position and not curved or arched. Draw your shoulders back so that your upper back is flat and not rounded. You should feel your stomach muscles working to stabilize you and a little tension between the shoulder blades throughout the exercise. Now, with your palm

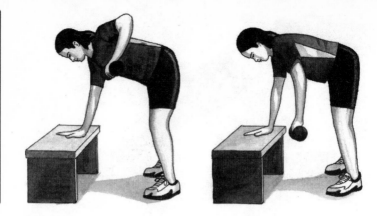

figure 16 the single arm row

facing behind you, simply bend your arm and raise the dumbbell to the side of your chest ensuring that your elbow lifts higher than the line of your body to ensure maximum work in the back area. Squeeze your shoulder blades together at the top of the movement and then lower the weight and repeat. As you lower the weight you are simply straightening your arm to keep your shoulders level at the bottom of the movement. Do not allow the weight to pull you out of position, just move slowly and with control.

Shoulder press

Why do it?

A great exercise to strengthen and shape your shoulders and arms.

How do I do it?

Stand with your feet shoulder-width apart with your toes pointing forwards and your knees slightly bent. Tighten up your stomach muscles so that your spine is in its neutral position and not curved forwards or arched backwards. Begin with a dumbbell in each hand positioned just above and in front of your shoulders with your palms facing forwards. Now simply extend your arms to raise the weights above your head in a narrow arc so that they meet above your head. Do not allow the weights to move further apart than shoulder width throughout the movement and do not lock out your elbows when your arms are extended.

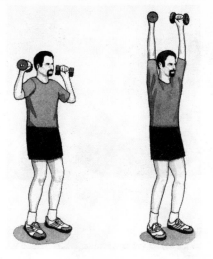

figure 17 the shoulder press

What are the options?

The exercise can be performed with your palms facing inwards if this is more comfortable. You can also do it sitting down but you must ensure that you sit upright supporting yourself with your stomach muscles rather than relying on the back of a chair to hold you upright.

Dumbbell flyes

Why do it?

A good exercise for strengthening the chest and shoulders while training the core stability muscles of the stomach.

How do I do it?

Lie face-up on a bench that is either flat or slightly inclined and raise a set of dumbbells above you. The weights should be above your chest rather than over your head with your elbows slightly bent and dumbbells end-on-end so your palms are facing towards your feet. Tighten up your stomach by drawing in your pelvic floor to ensure that your spine is in its neutral position. Maintain this stability throughout the exercise. Now, keeping a slight bend at the elbow, lower the weights slowly in a wide arc out to the side of your body until they are level with your shoulders. At the outermost point you will feel a stretch across

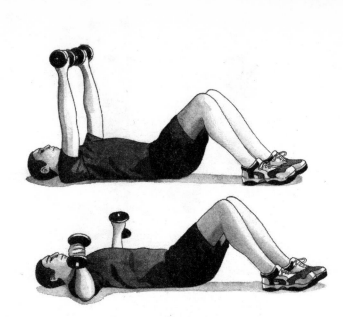

figure 18 the dumbbell fly

your chest. Return the weights to the starting position by squeezing the chest muscles, keeping the dumbbells over the chest. Try to keep the movement slow so that the lowering and raising phase take two seconds each. Do not bend your arms as this allows you to 'cheat' by using the biceps to move the weight.

What are the benefits?

For men this exercise helps to develop great pecs for the beach. For women it can be used to tone up and improve support around the bust area.

Pull over

Why do it?

This straightforward exercise works your back, shoulders, arms and stomach. It requires minimal equipment and is more

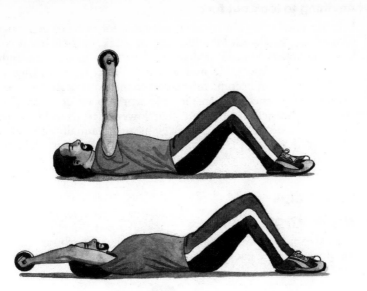

figure 19 the pull over

difficult than it looks if done properly, so engage the brain before taking it on.

How do I do it?

Lie on the floor with your knees bent and feet flat on the ground. Take a light weight – a dumbbell or substitute such as a large bottle of water – and hold it above your chest with your arms slightly bent at the elbows. Ensuring that you are stabilizing your body from the centre by contracting your stomach muscles (cough and then hold the tension in your belly, remember to breathe) slowly lower the weight over and behind your head towards the floor, keeping your elbows slightly bent. You will feel your shoulders and upper back working and there will come a point where you will feel the weight pulling your lower back off the floor. Work hard at the stomach to keep your back flat and then raise the weight slowly back to the vertical position. Do not bend your arms too much or you will work this area more than is necessary.

Anything to look out for?

Because your arms are straight there is a lot of force generated around the shoulder joint which can be weak, particularly if you have previously injured or dislocated it. Only move the weight as far as is comfortable and gradually increase the range of movement as you become more used to the exercise and you feel stronger. Also there is considerable work to be done by your abdominal muscles to prevent your lower back from lifting off the floor so begin with a light weight and gradually increase it but only if you can continue to hold a stable position in the lumbar area.

Bench dips

Why do it?

A good exercise for the major muscles of the upper body – chest, shoulders and the backs of your arms. Also good for livening up a run in the park.

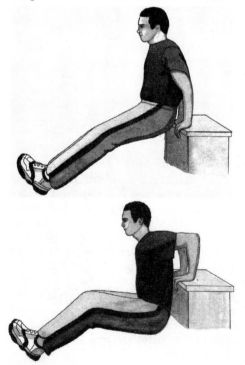

figure 20 the bench dip

How do I do it?

Sit on a bench with your hands next to your bottom and fingers pointing forwards. Extend your legs so that your feet are away from the bench and then lift yourself up so you are supported by your hands and feet. Now, keeping your bottom close to the bench, use your arms to lower your body towards the ground. Make sure that as your elbows bend, they point behind you and do not flap out to the sides. Your bottom should almost touch the ground and then, using your arms rather than your legs, raise yourself back up to the starting position. If you need to make the exercise more difficult you can move your feet further away from the bench but make sure that you keep your bottom close to the bench otherwise you will tend to push up with the legs rather than working the arms completely.

Shoulder raises

Why do it?

A great exercise to improve strength and definition of all the muscles of the shoulder.

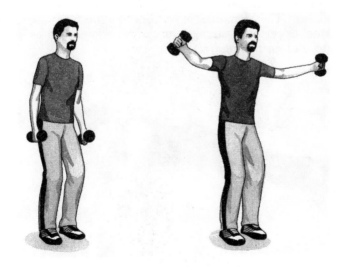

figure 21 the shoulder raise

How do I do it?

This exercise can be performed with dumbbells or with bottles of water if you do not have any exercise equipment to hand. Stand upright with your feet hip-width apart, knees slightly flexed, stomach held in to support you, and your shoulders back and down. Make sure that your scapula is relaxed and that you do not feel any tension in the upper back or neck. Your weights or water bottles should be held at your sides with your elbows slightly bent, your head in line with your body and not jutting forwards at the chin. Keeping a constant, slight bend at the elbows raise the weights out to the side and up to shoulder height. Pause at the top of the movement and then lower the weights back down to your sides slowly without letting gravity take over the movement. Always keep your palms facing down towards the floor. Make sure that you remain upright throughout the exercise. If you feel that you are bending at the waist slightly to lift the weights then you are probably using too much weight and so use a little less until you can perform the exercise correctly.

Press-up with hop

A more advanced version of a regular press-up for a really tough workout. The dynamic movement is good for generating 'elastic' upper body strength, useful for sports such as netball, rugby and for boxing training.

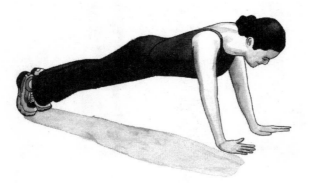

figure 22 the press-up with hop

Men

Prepare yourself for a regular press-up. Feet on the ground, hands shoulder-width apart, elbows slightly flexed, eyes to the ground slightly in front of you with your neck in line with your body and your scapula retraced so your shoulders are not rounded. Lower your chest to the floor and use the elasticity of the muscles to 'spring' out of this position with enough force to allow you to hop your hands off the ground at the top of the movement. Make sure you land with your elbows slightly flexed and then ease into the second press-up.

Women

Position yourself as above only have your knees in contact with the ground.

Variations

The exercise can be made more difficult by moving your hands closer together and made easier by moving them further apart. Whichever position you are in do not allow your shoulders to become rounded.

Tricep extension

Why do it?

An exercise which targets that hard-to-shift upper arm wobble and develops a lovely shape beneath the shoulders.

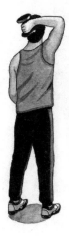

figure 23 the tricep extension

How do I do it?

Stand upright with your feet hip-width apart and your stomach muscles on to stabilize you. With a light dumbbell to begin with, raise one arm straight above your head, keeping good posture and not allowing your back to arch. Now lower the weight slowly behind your head by bending at the elbow but keeping your bicep close to your ear. Do not allow your elbow to drop down towards the floor. Take care not to lower the weight onto your head by rotating your shoulder so that the dumbbell can drop behind you. When your elbow is fully flexed you will feel a stretch in the back of your arm. Now straighten your arm above you without locking your elbow out at the top of the movement.

Bicep curls

Why do it?

Not just for muscle-heads but a good arm-toning exercise for men and women. Also a good functional exercise as you never know when you might need extra strength in your arms.

How do I do it?

Posture is all-important for this exercise and if you get it wrong you won't be exercising the bits you think you are. Take a

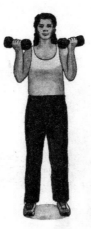

figure 24 the bicep curl

dumbbell in each hand and stand with your feet hip-width apart, knees slightly bent and toes forward. You should stand very tall with your neck extended and your shoulders back and down. Let the weights hang by your sides with your elbows slightly bent and tucked into the side of your body. Your palms should be facing the sides of your thighs. Take a moment to tighten up at the stomach so that you can hold your upright position while you move the weights and then bend at the elbow slowly to bring the dumbbells up towards your shoulders. As you raise the dumbbells gradually twist your wrists so that you end up with your palms facing your shoulders. Squeeze your biceps at the top of the movement and then lower the weights slowly, twisting your wrists back 90 degrees and keeping your elbows at your sides without allowing them to travel behind the line of your body.

Pull-ups

Why do it?

This is an exercise that is hard to do but, when done correctly, will give great results for your back and your biceps as well as giving your abdominal area a tough workout.

How do I do it?

First you need to find a low bar, which will most likely be a fence or piece of equipment in a children's playground – just make sure you do not upset any of the children. Sit underneath the bar and then take hold of it with a reverse grip so that your palms are towards you and knuckles facing away. Your hands

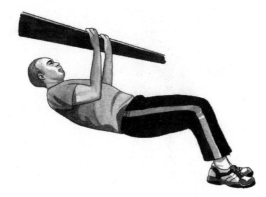

figure 25 the pull-up

should be slightly wider than shoulder-width apart. Now straighten your legs out in front of you and take your weight through your arms. You should now be dangling underneath the bar with your legs out, feet on the floor, and your chest directly below the bar. Take a moment to activate your stomach muscles for stability and pull back your shoulder blades so you are open at the chest and shoulders. Keeping your body in a straight line from shoulders to ankles, pull with your arms and back to raise your chest to the bar. Then lower your body keeping a slight bend at your elbows at the bottom of the movement, and making sure that you do not round your shoulders at any point.

This one is hard – is there an easy way to get started?

Bending your legs makes the exercise slightly easier so you may want to begin this way and gradually progress to completing sets with your legs fully extended in front of you.

Reverse flyes

Why do it?

A great exercise for strengthening the lower back and stomach while adding muscle to the mid-back area. This is important as too many people spend a lot of time exercising the 'mirror muscles' and neglecting those they cannot see. Do not forget that on the beach people can see the back of you as well as the front!

How do I do it?

Take light dumbbells to begin and stand with your feet hip-width apart. Bend at the knees and hips so that you are in a half-

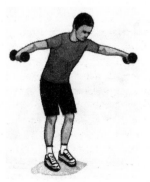

figure 26 the reverse fly

squat position with your upper body at 45 degrees to the ground. Allow the weights to dangle beneath you with your elbows bent slightly and your scapula retracted so your shoulders are flat to the ground and not rounded. Your lower back should also be flat or in its neutral position supported by your deep abdominal muscles. Now raise the weights out sideways slowly using the muscles of your back and rear shoulder. Do not swing them out to the side. At the top of the movement concentrate on squeezing your shoulder blades together and then lower the weights slowly.

Any other ways to do this one?

If you have a weak lower back you can still perform the exercise with light weights by sitting on a bench and leaning forwards, supporting your upper body on your thighs.

Abdominal/core training exercises

Abdominal curls

Why do it?

To strengthen the trunk area providing a great stable base for the rest of your exercise routine and as you move around in your daily life.

How do I do it?

Lie flat on your back with your knees bent and feet flat on the floor. Stabilize your low back by tightening the pelvic floor and then use your abdominal muscles to curl up at the waist and lift the shoulders from the floor. Your arms can be held across your chest or you can slide your hands up your thighs as you move. Keep your head in line with your body as if you had an orange between your chin and your chest. This will help you to keep your shoulders relaxed and will prevent any of the tension in the neck area that others sometimes feel when performing this exercise. Your pelvis and legs should not move while you lift the shoulders. Pause briefly at the top of the movement and then lower slowly without letting your head drop back to the floor. There should be no sharp movements or 'bouncing' during this exercise. The whole thing from start to finish should be controlled by your deep stomach muscles. Aim to breath out as you raise your shoulders making sure that you do not hold your breath at any stage.

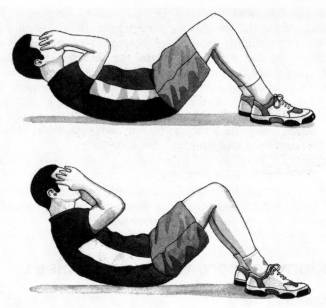

figure 27 the abdominal curl

Will I get a great six-pack?

A strong abdominal area is crucial for all activities and particularly important for protecting the lower back. Exercising this muscle area will help to tone your midriff but remember you will also have to burn off any excess fat hiding your six-pack with your regular routine of CV exercise.

Reverse crunch

Why do it?

Well worth adding to your routine as it has been shown to be the exercise that works the most muscles of the abdominal area in one movement.

How do I do it?

Lie on the floor, face up with your head and neck relaxed and your arms by your sides. Cough gently to tighten up your stomach muscles and then maintain this tension in the stomach and remember to breathe naturally. Now, stabilizing from the stomach so that your back remains flat on the ground, lift one foot off the floor and then the other so that your thighs are

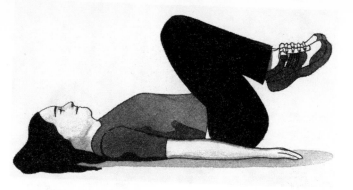

figure 28 the reverse crunch

perpendicular to the ground. Now, using your lower abdominal muscles, slowly draw your knees in towards your chest as far as you can, aiming to raise your bottom and lower back a little way off the floor. Then return to the starting position without letting your knees travel too far away from your body. If you feel your lower back arching up from the floor you have gone too far. You should always bring your knees back towards your chest before you begin to feel the exercise pulling on your lower back.

How does it fit into my routine?

Use this exercise as part of your overall stomach and low back workout to improve your core stability, balance and strength.

Double crunch

Why do it?

To work the whole of the abdominal area from deep down core stability muscles to the upper and lower sections of the more superficial 'six–pack' muscles.

How do I do it?

Lie on the floor face up with your knees bent and feet flat on the ground. Activate your deep stomach muscles by coughing and holding the tension and then carefully raise your feet, one at a time, off the ground so that you end up with both thighs perpendicular to the floor. This is your starting and finishing position. Now, with slow movements, regular breathing and consistent core stability, gently raise your shoulders off the

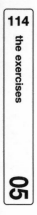

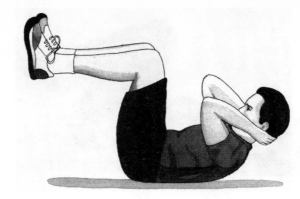

figure 29 the double crunch

ground while at the same time bringing your knees towards your chest. Pause briefly at the top of the movement and then lower slowly without losing tension in your deep stomach muscles. This will ensure that your lower back is not compromised. Repeat, keeping the movements slow so that you are working the muscles hard all the way through the set.

Twist crunch

Why do it?

An exercise to strengthen your core area and the sides of your stomach which are important for any sport that requires rotational movement such as tennis, netball, football, dancing and martial arts.

How do I do it?

Lie on the floor face up with your knees bent and feet flat and slightly apart. Breathe deeply to relax and then stabilize your low back by tightening your pelvic floor. Now use your abdominal muscles to curl up at the waist and lift the shoulders from the floor. Keep your head in line with your body as if you had an orange between your chin and your chest. Your pelvis and legs should not move while you lift the shoulders. At the top of the movement twist your shoulders to one side, keeping your head in line then return them to the centre position and lower without letting them touch the floor. Repeat the movement but this time twist your shoulders to the opposite side. When you have completed 10 twists to each side take a rest and then repeat the set.

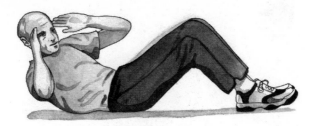

figure 30 the twist crunch

Anything to watch out for?

Make sure that at all times during the exercise your lower back and feet are flat on the ground. If either lift off the floor then you need to slow down the movement and control it from your stomach.

The plank

Why do it?

An exercise that improves abdominal strength without putting strain on the lower back. It also provides a good alternative to traditional stomach crunches and sit-ups.

How do I do it?

Lie face down on the floor with your arms bent so that they are underneath you and you are supported on your elbows. Now tighten up your stomach muscles and raise your hips off the floor far enough to create a straight line from your shoulders to your knees which are still in contact with the ground. Be careful not to let your hips sag so that your back arches. Similarly do not raise your hips too high so that the exercise becomes easy. Hold this position for 8–10 seconds and then relax. Make sure that you keep breathing as you hold the position – holding your breath will only lead to a rise in blood pressure. Repeat this 8 times making sure you hold the position steady on each effort.

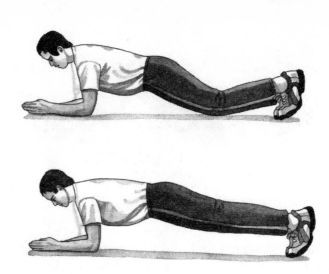

figure 31 the plank

What if I want to make it more difficult?

To make the exercise more difficult you can start in the same position but raise both your hips and your knees at the same time so you are balancing on your elbows and toes/balls of your feet with your body in a straight line from shoulders to ankles. If you need more of a challenge raise one foot off the ground while you hold the position. Alternate legs and gradually increase the duration of the hold.

Hip lift bridge

Why do it?

To develop strength and stability in the bottom and abdomen.

How do I do it?

Lie on the floor face up and bend your knees so that you can place your feet flat on the ground. Tighten up your pelvic floor so your abdominal area feels firm and your back is in a neutral (straight) position. Now slowly raise your hips until you have a straight line from your knees to your shoulders and then hold this position. Squeeze your buttock cheeks together to hold the

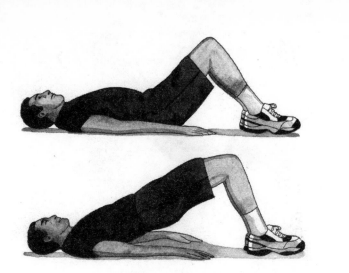

figure 32 the hip lift bridge

position steady. Do not let your hips sag or arch them too much so that you feel pain in the lower back. Your aim is to complete 5–10 repetitions of the exercise holding each one for as long as you can.

Why is it important?

Many sports, running for example, can put an excessive strain on the hamstrings whilst leaving the bottom muscles weak. This bridging exercise encourages your core area and bottom to work together to stabilize your body, leaving your hamstrings free to move you.

Flexibility training exercises

Hamstring stretch

Why do it?

Many people spend a lot of their time sitting down which means that their hamstrings – located at the back of the thighs – can

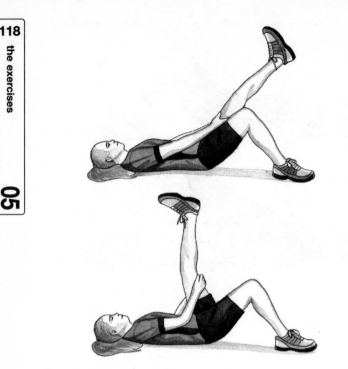

figure 33 the hamstring stretch

become shortened over time. A long-term result of this is that the hamstrings may become tight and unable to fully extend which can cause misalignment of the pelvis and lower back. Stretching your hamstrings regularly will stop them becoming short and could prevent issues such as back pain in the future.

How do I do it?

Lie face up with your knees bent and feet flat on the floor. Lift one leg and straighten it above you but do not lock out the knee joint. Keeping the leg straight clasp your hands at the back of the knee joint and pull the leg gently towards your chest until you feel a stretch at the back of the thigh. Hold this position for 8–10 seconds and then release the leg slowly. Follow the sequence for the other leg and then repeat for both legs.

Is there anything particular to look out with on this one?

Do not stretch too suddenly but move gradually to the point where you feel mild tension in the muscle being stretched. Do not bounce into a stretch, simply hold and release, and never stretch a cold muscle – always ensure that you have thoroughly warmed up before you stretch any part of your body.

Glute stretch

Why do it?

The muscles of your bottom are used a great deal every day – and not just for sitting on. This stretch will help keep them in good condition.

How do I do it?

Lie on your back with your knees bent and feet flat on the ground. Cross your right leg over your left so that your right ankle sits just above your left knee and allow your right knee to relax towards the floor. Tighten your stomach muscles and lift your left foot off the floor far enough to allow you to clasp your hands behind your left thigh. Now draw your arms in to pull the left leg towards you while keeping the right leg relaxed. As your

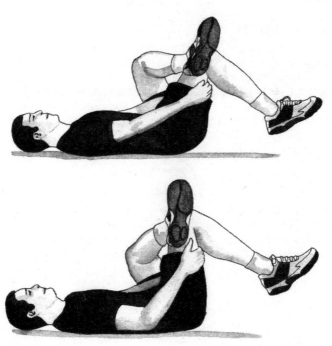

figure 34 the glute stretch

legs come nearer your chest you should feel a stretch in the right side of your bottom. Do not overdo it but move into the stretch slowly and then hold for 8–10 seconds. Then repeat the process for the other leg.

Are these muscles important?

When you stand, walk around or participate in sports, the muscles of your bottom, your gluteal muscles, should be used to stabilize your hips and help protect your lower back. This means that they have to work hard and can become tight. By stretching them regularly you can maintain the elasticity in the muscles and help prevent injury in this area.

Quad stretch

Why do it?

The muscles at the front of your thighs get a tough workout when running, cycling, stepping or trampolining. If they become tight, even walking can become painful which can seriously affect your day and is to be avoided at all costs.

How do I do it?

Stand up straight close to a wall or chair you can use for support. Keep one foot on the ground with the knee of this leg slightly bent. Bring the heel of the other foot up towards your bottom by bending the leg at the knee. Grab onto the foot of

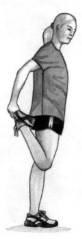

figure 35 the quad stretch

your bent leg. Keeping your knees together, push forwards at the hip of your fully bent leg and you will feel a stretch radiating along the front of this thigh. To increase the stretch bring the foot closer to your bottom and push this hip slightly further forwards. Slowly relax out of the stretch and repeat for the other leg.

Inner thigh stretch

Why do it?
You often see people stretching out their thighs, calves and hamstrings but the insides of the legs are often overlooked. But as they are muscles that are used whenever you are moving around and they stop your legs from flying out sideways from underneath you, you ignore them at your peril.

How do I do it?
A simple way to stretch out the entire inner thigh area is to sit on the floor with your feet wide apart and your hands behind you for support. Be sure to activate your deep stomach muscles for core stability so that your back is neutral and your pelvis is in the optimum position for this stretch. Now simply push your body forwards with your hands so that your feet move gradually further apart under control. The further you move the more of a stretch you will feel. Hold the position for 10–15 seconds and then you will probably feel the stretch ease off a little. Now you can move slightly further forwards for maximum stretching and because you are in a comfortable seated position you can hold the stretch for as long as you like.

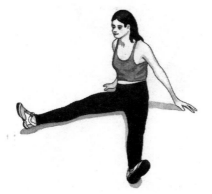

figure 36 the inner thigh stretch

Back and hamstring stretch

Why do it?

Getting into this position provides a really good stretch for the lower back and for the hamstrings, particularly the muscles running down the outside of the back of the leg. It is especially good for anyone who usually just stretches the centre of the hamstrings and those who regularly feel tightness in their back.

How do I do it?

Lie on the floor face up with your shoulders flat on the floor and your knees bent to about 45 degrees. Keeping your shoulder blades on the floor, allow your knees to roll over to one side making sure that your knees and feet stay together. This might be enough of a movement to give you a stretch in the lower back. Extend the top leg and, keeping the leg straight, bring the foot up towards your head. Now, with your body as still as you can keep it, lock out the knee of the upper leg. In this position you should feel quite an acute stretch behind the kneecap of the straight leg. The stretch should radiate up the leg, around the bottom and into the back.

> **WARNING** This exercise should be done slowly and with control from your abdominal muscles. If you feel pain in your lower back at any stage you should stop immediately.

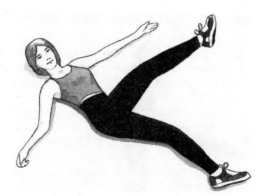

figure 37 the back and hamstring stretch

Cat and dog stretch

Why do it?

This exercise is very useful for anyone who has a tight back or who is at risk from developing back problems due to long bouts of sitting at a desk or in the car.

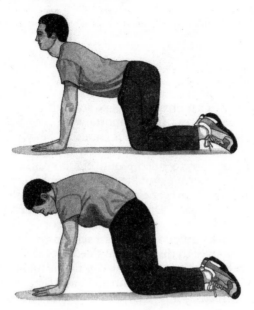

figure 38 the cat and dog stretch

How do I do it?

Adopt a position on the floor where you are on your hands and knees with a secure and balanced posture – shoulders should be over hands and hips over knees. Now relax your stomach so that it falls towards the floor whilst at the same time lifting your head and arching your bottom outwards behind you so that you feel your spine is as extended as it can be along its length. You will feel this part of the exercise primarily as a stretch in the lower back. Now drop your head and pull your stomach in gradually, moving through the point where your torso is parallel with the ground and then drop your head, suck your tummy in and make your back as round as you can. Imagine a piece of string between your shoulder blades that is being pulled up towards the ceiling. You should feel this part of the movement as a stretch in the mid and upper back. Hold this position for 5 seconds and return slowly to the arching position. Repeat both parts of the stretch 5 times and then relax.

Knee rolls

Why do it?

For all those who feel tightness in the lower back, this simple exercise can be a source of great relief.

How do I do it?

Lie on the floor face up with your knees bent and feet flat and together. Take a deep breath to relax yourself and then tighten up your stomach area. It is important to feel that you are controlling this exercise from your stomach. Slowly lower your legs to one side keeping your knees and feet together by allowing the top foot to ride up onto the bottom one. As your legs drop to the side your shoulder blades should stay flat on the floor and, as your knees get close to the floor, you should feel a stretch in the lower back. Drop the knees over as far as they will go and hold the lowest position for a few seconds. With control from the stomach bring your knees back up to the centre and then drop them over to the opposite side. Repeat the movement 5 times to each side. As you repeat you might find that you are able to lower your legs slightly further each time as your back loosens up. Practise this exercise as often as possible for optimum back mobility.

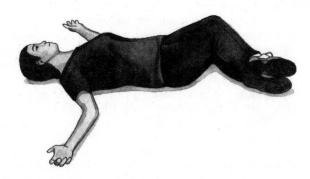

figure 39 the knee roll

Upper back stretch

Why do it?

To help ease out those muscles through the upper and middle back.

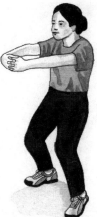

figure 40 the upper back stretch

How do I do it?

Stand with your feet hip-width apart and your knees slightly bent. Clasp your hands together in front of your chest with your palms facing your body and then move your hands forwards until your elbows are bent to around 90 degrees. Now move your hands forwards without changing the angle at your elbows which means you have to move forwards at the shoulders. This lengthens the muscles between your spine and your shoulders and gives your back a very satisfying stretch.

Chest stretch

Why do it?

This stretch will help to balance the effects of sitting over a desk all day.

How do I do it?

If your shoulders are hunched forwards too often, your chest muscles may become shortened. To redress this imbalance, clasp your hands behind your body with your palms just behind your

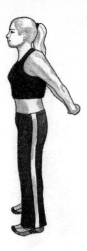

figure 41 the chest stretch

bottom. Gently lift your hands slowly away from your bottom while at the same time squeezing your shoulder blades together. This will allow your chest and shoulders to open at the front of your body. Keep your shoulders relaxed throughout this stretch to avoid feeling tension around the neck area.

Tricep stretch

Why do it?

Repeated use of the muscles at the back of the arm can leave them tight which can impair movement above your head. Stretching this area will keep it supple and maintain full movement.

How do I do it?

Stand upright with your shoulders relaxed. Raise your left arm above your head and bend the elbow so that your forearm moves down behind your head until your hand rests at the nape of your neck. Use your right hand to increase the movement by gently pulling your left elbow further behind your head. Relax slowly out of the movement and repeat on the other side.

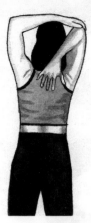

figure 42 the tricep stretch

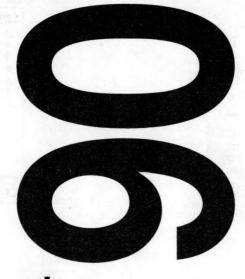

06

taking action

In this chapter you will learn:
- how to structure your first workout
- how to complete your first workout
- how to progress your fitness programme.

Before we go any further, here is a reminder of some essential advice for your training programme.

General training tips

Good posture is essential both for exercising safely and for working the parts of your body that you are intending to work. If your posture is poor, your body will be misaligned and you may end up exercising muscles in a way that may not achieve the results you are aiming for, or could lead to injury. This applies to CV exercise, strength training and flexibility work. Always engage your deep stomach muscles to stabilize your lower back area and protect your spine. The easiest way to do this is to contract your pelvic floor, sit or stand up straight, pull your shoulders slightly back and down and lift your head by imagining a string pulling you upwards from the crown of your head.

If your chosen CV exercise involves your whole body – running, cross training, stepping, stair running – **get your whole body involved** and burn maximum calories by working your arms as vigorously as you work your legs. If you choose to swim, ensure your legs are working hard and that you are not relying only on your arms to propel you.

Monitor your effort level by using a simple rating scale of one to ten. Two out of ten may be anything slightly more strenuous than a gentle walk. Nine out of ten is the point where you are ready to drop. By using the scale you will be able to judge the value of each of your workouts and predict the speed of your results. The more often you work at the top end of the scale, the quicker your progress will be.

Breathe deeply. Your lungs are more efficient the more you use them. Getting air deep into your lungs allows more oxygen to get to the working muscles more quickly which will bring you faster fitness gains and improved stamina.

You can determine the specific effects a strength training programme will have on your body if you **select the correct weights** and the optimum number of sets and repetitions for your needs. With any new exercise, begin by using a light weight until you are comfortable with the movement and you can perform the exercise with good posture and good technique. Gradually increase the weight until you are only able to do 20 repetitions and no more.

When you are confident with the technique of an exercise you can **decide on the results you want**. Sets of 20 will tone your muscles, sets of 15 will sculpt them and sets of 10–12 will achieve optimum strength gains. When selecting your programmes and your desired results, choose a weight that ensures the number of repetitions you are performing is the maximum you are able to do. If you are aiming to tone the backs of your arms, choose a weight that means 20 repetitions of the tricep extension is the most you can do before you need to rest. If you could do more than 20 your progress will be more gradual. For quickest results, choose a heavier weight as soon as you feel confident doing so.

Stay hydrated during all your workouts. The best way to do this is to drink water steadily throughout every day in order that you are well hydrated when you begin your exercise session. Sip water regularly as you exercise and then keep drinking, roughly half a litre, during the 30–60 minutes following your workout.

Stretches should be performed slowly to avoid pulling muscles suddenly into positions in which they are uncomfortable. Each stretch should be held for 8–10 seconds, with concentrated attention on the area being stretched. If you cannot feel the stretch properly, adjust your position until you can. If any area is particularly tight, hold these stretches for longer and perform them more often throughout the day.

Suggested exercise programmes

The objective of this book is that you will fully understand how to *Teach Yourself Fitness*. The suggested programmes are starting points to help you move in the direction of discovering what programme of exercise will work for you and bring you the specific results you are looking for. There are a number of exercises to choose from so if there are some you would specifically like to try, put these into your programme instead of some of the suggestions. The most important thing is that you make a start on finding our how *you* can fit exercise into *your* life, what type of exercise you enjoy the most, and how quickly you can get the best results. By using the feedback from your diary, you will have all the information you need for your optimum fitness plan. Your diary should be kept up to date at all times and used throughout your fitness life. It is the essential tool for monitoring your success and speeding up your progress.

Programme 1 will get you started with your exercise. It can be performed in the gym or with weights at home. Choose weights that ensure 20 repetitions is the most you can do for each strength training exercise. Feel free to swap the walking warm-up and CV training section for other options of your choice, maybe trampolining, skipping or cycling.

Programme 1	Exercise	Time/Intensity
Warm-up	Fast Walking	3 minutes
CV training	Running	10 minutes
Strength training	Squats	1 x 20
	Press-ups	1 x 20
	Single arm row	1 x 20
	Shoulder press	1 x 20
	Lunges	1 x 20
Core training	Reverse crunch	1 x 20
	Hip lift bridge	x 5
Flexibility training	Hamstring Stretch	Hold all stretches
	Glute Stretch	for 8–10 seconds
	Knee Rolls	
	Quad Stretch	
	Chest Stretch	
	Upper Back Stretch	

Aim to complete programme 1 two to three times each week for a period of four weeks. Note down all your progress, results and emotions in your exercise diary.

Programme 2 will increase the intensity of your workout and suggests a way of working that is time efficient and will keep your heart rate up and your muscles challenged. Move on to programme 2 when you feel you have learnt from programme 1, obtained the feedback you need from completing it, and you feel you are ready for a new challenge.

Interval training

CV interval training involves working yourself to different levels of exertion within one workout. For example, once you have warmed up, you may exercise at a high intensity for 30 seconds and then recover for 90 seconds. The physical benefits of interval training are that by increasing your heart rate and exertion level during the tough intervals, you will burn more calories and create greater fitness improvements during the easier intervals than you would if you simply started exercising at this lower level and remained here throughout your workout.

The mental benefits of interval training are that you will be able to work much harder if you think the higher exertion level is only for 30 seconds or a similar short period of time than if you try to work this hard for the whole workout. Any workout with interval training also seems to pass much faster than a session of steady state training. Instead of watching the clock and counting down the seconds to the end as you can do when you are working at one level, with interval training you are either willing the time to pass slowly on your recovery phases or are so preoccupied with working hard in the tough sections that you need to focus on your body and breathing rather than the time.

Interval training is a great way to progress your fitness quickly and, to begin with, you only need small changes in the intensity level to see a big difference in your performance. As you become more comfortable with this way of training, you can increase the difference in exertion level between the tough sections and the recovery sections. You can do this by making the tough intervals harder or longer, or by reducing the amount of recovery time you have between each period of high intensity exercise.

Altering the terrain while running or cycling is a form of interval training as pushing yourself uphill will naturally make you work harder.

For programme 2, interval training should be performed alternating periods of one minute high intensity and one minute recovery. For example, once you have completed your warm-up, run for one minute at a level you feel is a six out of ten effort, then for one minute at a level you feel is an eight out of ten effort. Repeat this pattern five times. As with programme 1, if you prefer to use a different form of CV exercise, feel free to do so but follow the same guidelines for your interval training.

Strength training should be performed in a circuit by working through one set of 15 for each exercise in order and then repeating a second set of each exercise. Choose weights that ensure 15 repetitions is the most you can complete for each set of each strength training exercise.

Aim to complete programme 2 two to three times each week for a period of four weeks. Note down all your progress, results and emotions in your exercise diary.

Programme 2	Exercise	Time/Intensity
Warm-up	Running – moderate	3 minutes
CV training	Running – intervals	10 minutes
Strength training	Lunges	1 x 15 reps of each
	Bench dips	exercise and then
	Single arm row	repeat the
	Squat jumps	sequence
	Tricep extensions	
	Bicep curls	
Core training	Abdominal curls	1 x 15
	Twist crunch	1 x 15
Flexibility training	Hamstring stretch	Hold all stretches
	Glute stretch	for 8–10 seconds
	Cat and Dog stretch	
	Quad stretch	
	Chest stretch	
	Upper back stretch	

Programme 3 suggests a further way of structuring your workout. Use programme 3 when you have mastered programme 2 and have learnt all you need to from it.

CV training for programme 3 should be performed with stepped increments: one minute high intensity, one minute recovery and one minute moderate intensity. These stepped increments allow you to gradually work harder through each 'step' as your body becomes accustomed to the exertion, allowing you to push on a little bit harder for the next stage. You may need to experiment a little with the levels you use for each step and with practice you will be able to structure a workout on each piece of CV kit that will enable you to reach maximum effort level by the end of your time on each machine.

Strength Training in programme 3 should be performed with exercises in pairs. Complete one set of the first exercise, then the first set of the second, the second set of the first exercise and then the second set of the second exercise. This allows you to keep rests to a minimum and work yourself hard throughout your session. Choose weights that ensure 12 repetitions is the most you can complete for each set of each strength training exercise.

Aim to complete programme 3 two to three times each week for a period of four weeks. Note down all your progress, results and emotions in your exercise diary.

Programme 3	Exercise	Time/Intensity
Warm-up	Skipping – moderate	3 minutes
CV training	Skipping – stepped intervals	12 minutes
Strength training	{ Wide leg squats { Shoulder raises	1 x 12
	{ Lunges { Pull-ups	
	{ Pull over { Press-up with hop	
	{ Lunge jumps { Shoulder press	
Core training	Reverse crunch	x 15
	Double crunch	x 15
	The plank	Hold for 8 seconds x 5
Flexibility training	Hamstring stretch	Hold all stretches for 8–10 seconds
	Glute stretch	
	Chest stretch	
	Triceps stretch	
	Upper back stretch	
	Back/hamstring stretch	

What do I do next?

Once you have tried all three programmes and recorded your results, thoughts and feedback in your diaries, you will be in a position to plan your own specific fitness routine with full knowledge of the exercises you like, what works most effectively for you, what keeps you interested and the times and days when exercise best fits into your schedule. Chapter 7 will show you how to put all this information together. Begin here by outlining your initial thoughts on what you would like to do.

My personal fitness programme	Exercise	Time/Intensity
Warm-up		
CV training		
Strength training		
Core training		
Flexibility training		

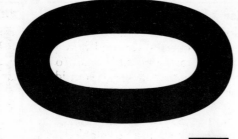

07 designing your own personal fitness programme

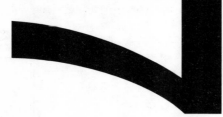

In this chapter you will learn:
- how to create your personal fitness programme
- how to design your personal fitness checklist
- how to progress your own personal fitness programme.

Fitness goals

Now that exercise has become part of your life, it is time to focus specifically on what really works for you and how you will get the results you want in the shortest possible time. To do this, first remind yourself of your objectives. Some of your ideas may have evolved since you thought about them in earlier chapters, and that's fine. You now have more knowledge of exercise and how you feel about it, so use this knowledge to develop your thoughts and make them more attainable. Let's pick out some key questions from earlier and note down your up-to-date answers.

What is my one key fitness aim?

....

By what date will I have achieved this goal?

....

What will I do to ensure I reach my goal?

....

List three other fitness priorities.

....

....

....

Are my objectives all specific, measurable, achievable, realistic and time-framed?

....

Do I have all the resources I need?

....

Can I visualize myself achieving my objectives?

....

Do I have the knowledge, the motivation and the correct timing to ensure success?

....

Once you have the answers to the above questions, you will be mentally ready to prepare your personal fitness plan. Here is an example of a plan created by one individual after she answered the questions above.

My personal fitness programme – Katherine, February 2005

Fitness goals

- To continue with my swimming x 1 per week.
- To structure a format for my swimming training.
- To continue with my Aerobics session x 1 per week.
- To incorporate some strength training that will help me with my running.
- To restore running as part of my weekly training session.
- To complete a formally organized 10 km run on 4 April 2005.
- To run the race without walking breaks.
- To complete the race in approximately one hour.
- I must complete the entry form for the race before the end of February 2005.

Here we can see some clear objectives with a strong focus on where this exercise programme is headed. Let's now look at what Katherine came up with for the overview of her schedule.

Cardiovascular training

Aerobics class: Once a week on Wednesday evening

Swim training: Once a week on Friday morning

Running: Once a week, long run on Saturday morning

Running: Once a week interval, sprint or hill training session on Monday evening

Strength training

All exercises to be completed once per week. Strength training day will be determined at the beginning of each week depending on work, travel and family schedule.

Two sets of 20 reps of each exercise to be performed

Squats, Lunges, Lunge jumps, Squat jumps, Single-leg squats

Posture exercises

Practise good core stability from the abdominals and glutes at all times.

Always keep shoulders back and down allowing arms to move freely.

Keep good spinal alignment, with particular attention to head on top of shoulders, not jutting out in front.

And now let's look at the details for Katherine's exercise sessions

Exercise programmes – Katherine

Swimming	Distance	Intensity
30 Minutes	Warm-up x 4 lengths 2 lengths 1 length Repeat x 6 Cool down x 2 lengths	Easy breast stroke Front crawl Breast stroke Easy breast stroke

Swimming	Distance	Intensity
Progression	Warm-up x 4 lengths 3 lengths 1 length Repeat x 6 Cool down x 2 lengths	Easy breast stroke Front crawl Breast stroke Easy breast stroke

Running	Time/Distance	Intensity
Sprint training	Warm-up x 5 minutes 200 m 200 m Repeat x 4 Cool-down x 3 minutes	Easy jog Sprint Recovery/jog Easy jog

Running	Time/Distance	Intensity
Sprint training Progression	Warm-up x 5 minutes 400 m 400 m Repeat x 4 Cool-down x 3 minutes	Easy jog Sprint Recovery/jog Easy jog

Running	Time	Progression
Long run	30 minutes	Increase run by at least 2 minutes each time

Weekly fitness checklist

To help Katherine stay on track, she used a simple checklist to monitor how everything stacked up during the week. The results of the checklist were used in conjunction with her exercise diary to refine the approach. You can devise your own checklist and simply tick each box as you complete each workout to keep you on track from week to week.

Here is how Katherine's checklist looked:

Week	Monday Sprints	Wednesday Aerobics	Friday Swim	Saturday Long Run	Day TBC Strength training
1					
2					
3					
4					
5					
6					
7					
8					
9					
10					

Katherine's main objective was to complete her 10 km run which she successfully did, and within her target time. On 5 April, following her success, she embarked on an updated fitness plan with new objectives. This is key to always moving forwards with fitness and if you stick to this pattern of continually updating what you want out of your fitness programme, you will be successful, now and forever in the future.

You can design as many programmes for yourself as you like – there is a template you can use in the appendix of this book, or you can format your own way of recording your workouts. By using your workouts in conjunction with your diary you will always know which programme to use in order to achieve specific results at any given time.

There is also a template in the appendix for devising your own personal fitness checklist. Always use your checklist and your exercise diary to make adjustments to your fitness programme. Be completely honest with your assessment of your progress in order to get the best results. If your workouts are not getting done, you may need to rethink your schedule and your checklist. If you are beginning to find workouts easier or your progress is slow, you need to note this down and take the appropriate action by increasing the duration of your CV workout or the intensity of your strength training. If you are not enjoying your exercise, or you are finding your workouts dull and uninspiring, record this information and take steps to fix the situation.

Overcoming fitness boredom or a training plateau

Top tips

- Go for a short, sharp workout – decrease your rest periods, either between sets of repetitions or between different exercises.
- Change the number of repetitions per set or the total number of exercises you do in a session.
- Try a different piece of kit for your CV workout.
- Alter the speed of your run, bike ride or row.
- Change the order in which you do your exercises.
- Change the exercise for each muscle group. Do press-ups instead of dips, squats instead of lunges, dumbbell flys instead of single arm rows, single leg squats instead of wide leg squats.
- Create a circuit of exercises and quickly move from one to the next without resting between them.
- Select ten strength training exercises for a workout and complete three-minutes of high intensity CV blast between each exercise.

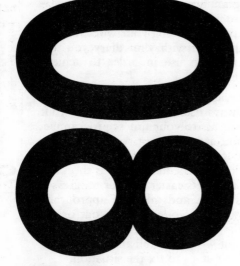

08 designing your own personal food plan

In this chapter you will learn:
- how to get started with your food plan
- what changes to make initially
- how to refine your food plan for long-term success.

Food is simple and you should aim to keep your food plan simple. The objective of your food diary is to enable you to track your eating plan, the plan that gives you your current results, and then make changes directed towards the results you really want.

Your food diary and the changes you make are very personal things but often people get stuck with where to start or what new ideas may work for them to achieve more positive results than their current plan. To help you get started, we will use the sample day's food diary referred to in Chapter 4 with some suggestions of new approaches and different types of food you can incorporate into your plan. Beyond this, it is up to you to determine changes that will cater for your tastes and your lifestyle, and will benefit your specific situation. The real value of using the food diary is that you are open to experimenting and having some fun with it.

It is worth trying as many different approaches as you can in order to discover what works best for you. The answer may not present itself immediately but stick with it and keep careful notes so that you can recognize when you are onto something. You may not need a major overhaul of your current eating pattern so take care to maintain what is working and complement it with other positive steps.

Give yourself a fair chance of finding the right pattern for your life. A particular meal or snack idea may not work immediately but be flexible in your approach and be prepared to try strategies at different times. Just as timing is important for finding your motivation to make general changes to your life, it is also important when making each of the changes in your diet so try all your strategies under a variety of different circumstances before giving up on them and moving on to try new ones. You may end up with different strategies for weekdays and weekends, or different strategies for when working in the office or when travelling, or for when at home and when on holiday. It does not matter how many different approaches you have, what matters is that you put the successful ones into action at the right times.

Let's remind ourselves of our sample daily food diary and then look at it in detail.

Sample daily eating diary – Ray

Day/Date/ Time	Food/Meal/ Drink	Hunger Rating (0-10)	Moods/Thoughts/ Observations
Mon 8 November			
10.30 a.m.	Coffee and muffin	10	Monday morning, terrible journey to work, needed something comforting
11.00 a.m.	Glass of water		
1.30 p.m.	Chicken sandwich crisps, apple	6	My usual lunch, enjoyed it, felt good afterwards
2.30 p.m. & 6.00 p.m.	Glass of water		
3.30 p.m.	Cup of tea and two biscuits	7	Felt a bit tired so had something to pep me up
9.30 p.m.	Two glasses of wine Pasta, chicken, pesto sauce, bit of salad. Cheesecake	10	Finished work late so felt a bit rushed but happy that I managed to knock this meal together despite it being quite late
11.00 p.m.	Cup of tea	1	Need my bedtime cuppa

What to look out for first

Ray's first meal of the day is at 10.30 a.m. so we need to look at the **timing** of food throughout the diary. If Ray gets up at 10.00 a.m., then breakfast at 10.30 a.m. is fine. We can find out specifically what time he does get up by questioning him further but, judging by the fact that he has arrived at work by the time he has his first meal, we can assume he'll have been up for probably a couple of hours and that is a couple of hours with the body running on empty, with **energy levels** at their lowest. No wonder he is looking for some comfort food by the time he has arrived at the office.

Ray has his first drink of water at 11.00 a.m. which will go some way towards keeping him **hydrated,** but after a night's sleep and a coffee at 10.30 a.m., one glass may not be enough.

Lunch at 1.30 p.m. looks pretty good. It is three hours since breakfast and the content of the meal is a mixture of protein with the chicken, carbohydrates with the bread, and fruit with the apple. The quality of this meal to Ray is reflected in the fact that he felt good afterwards but then he should have known he would as this meal appears to be tried and tested as part of his daily lunch **habit**. We can also question the role of the crisps in this daily habit and whether or not they would be missed if they were taken away or substituted with something more healthy and nutritious.

Ray has another couple of glasses of water during the afternoon and the evening, though there are also two cups of tea and two glasses of wine which will all counteract the benefits of the water by dehydrating his body.

Once the energy provided by lunch has been used up, Ray reaches for a hot drink and some biscuits to get him going again. This looks like part of a daily routine and Ray's diary for the rest of the week will tell us how often this pattern occurs. If it is a daily routine, we need to establish if it is in keeping with Ray's aims, or contrary to them. He can then decide how often during a week he would like the tea and biscuits to be a feature and what his alternatives for other days will be.

From 3.30 p.m. there is a long gap until the evening meal at 9.30 p.m.. This means eight-hours of working and moving around for Ray, fuelled only by tea, biscuits and water during the afternoon. This will undoubtedly leave him feeling sluggish and very hungry into the early evening. Feeling hungry means he is looking for something sweet to provide some quick energy and a couple of glasses of wine fit the bill perfectly to quickly boost the blood sugar levels.

Ray's evening meal looks good, particularly as he reports that he's pleased with himself for managing to cook something. The suggestion here is that, at this late hour, he could be tempted to heat up something processed or order a take-out meal, so this is positive. Once again, keeping the diary over a full week will show how often cooking appears in Ray's schedule and how often he opts for an easier alternative.

The diary is rounded off with a cup of tea as part of Ray's ritual of drawing a line under the day and shutting down for the night.

What to look for next

Let's take a look at the **variety** in Ray's food for this sample diary day. During this day, he eats:

- A muffin
- Chicken
- Bread
- Crisps
- An apple

- Biscuits
- Pasta
- Pesto sauce
- Salad
- Cheesecake

And he drinks:

- Coffee
- Tea

- Water
- Wine

That makes a total of 14 items. Now let's divide the items up into natural and whole-foods versus man-made and processed items.

Natural

- Chicken
- Apple

- Salad
- Water

Processed

- Muffin
- Bread
- Crisps
- Biscuits
- Pasta

- Pesto
- Cheesecake
- Coffee
- Tea
- Wine

Natural v. man-made – why does it matter?

As we discussed in Chapter 4, we should all aim to eat as many foods that give us energy as we can, and avoid those that rob us of energy as often as possible. Dividing the list up like this makes it very clear what we need more of, and what we need less of. Try it with the food on your diary and see how it all stacks up.

List all the food and drink you consume during a sample day's food diary:

147
designing your own
personal food plan

08

My sample day's food intake	My sample day's drink intake

Now divide the items into natural whole-foods versus processed food.

My sample day's food and drink intake – Natural	My sample day's food and drink intake – Processed

What can we do to change things?

Success with making food changes hinges on making simple changes gradually. If you try to overhaul everything in a major way all at once, it can become confusing and difficult to keep track of what is working and what is not. By taking a step-by-step approach you are always in control and you are always moving forwards. Even if you make only one change each week, you will still be making 52 changes to your food intake in a year which could make an enormous difference to your fitness, your body shape and your life.

So give yourself time to incorporate changes into your diet gradually and do not feel you have to fix everything overnight.

The changes you decide to make first are entirely dependent on how your food diary looks. Some suggestions for changes Ray could make are listed below. Some of them may be relevant for you too. If not, use the suggested changes as a guideline and consider similar strategies that you could use.

Suggested change 1

Eat earlier in the day. Start as you mean to go on by giving your body some nutrients and some energy for the day ahead. Eating at this point in the day gets the metabolism going and enables your body to function efficiently and burn fat calories effectively. Have at least one glass of water with whatever you choose for breakfast.

What are my options?

- Whole-grain cereal
- Muesli
- Fresh fruit
- Low fat yoghurt
- Whole-grain toast
- Smoothie
- Porridge
- Poached egg

Suggested change 2

Drink water steadily throughout the day. Staying hydrated will improve all functions in the body and keep energy levels high.

How will I manage that?

- Buy a two-litre bottle of water every day, or refill a bottle each day, and work your way through it gradually.

- If you have a water cooler, set an alarm, either a mental note or a reminder on your watch, phone or computer to ensure that you go and fill your glass regularly.
- If you are on the move, drink water where you can. Have some in your bag, in your car, and always drink water when in meetings or if you stop during your day to have a break.
- Drink at least one glass of water for every cup of tea, coffee or fizzy drink that you consume.

Suggested change 3

With a more nutritious start to the day, there is less chance of needing a sugar and caffeine hit mid-morning so go for something that will give you a slower energy release and more sustained energy.

What are my options?
- Fresh fruit
- Dried fruit
- Chopped vegetables with or without a healthy humous or tatziki dip
- Rice cakes
- Oat cakes
- Nuts

Suggested change 4

Plan ahead and do some shopping. You will have a pretty good idea of where you are going to be from week to week. So you will also know where the danger points are in your schedule where you might make poor food choices, perhaps because there is nothing healthy available. Planning your shopping carefully will mean that you will always have healthy options around.

How do I do that?
- Examine your weekly schedule and work out exactly where you are going to be each day.
- Think about what food choices will be available to you and plan your best options.
- If there are points looming in the week where there will be no healthy options or no food available at all, go shopping in

advance so you have something to get you through these moments.

- Always have something available that you like to snack on. There should be something healthy available in your desk and you should always have something in the fridge or the cupboard at home that you can grab in the morning to see you through any likely danger period in the day.

Suggested change 5

Prepare as much of your own food as you can. Buying and eating pre-packed and pre-prepared food means you are putting your dietary health in someone else's hands as you have no control what goes into these products.

What can I do instead?

- Buy enough food each week to ensure you have plenty of ingredients at home
- Prepare the equivalent of what you might buy ready made. It is not complicated, it won't take much longer, it will be cheaper and it will taste much nicer.
- Make snacks at home and take them with you. This may take a little time but probably less time than it would take you to run out and buy the same snack later. It will definitely save you money.

Make a concerted effort to incorporate at least two of these changes into your food diary within two weeks and then monitor the results. How do you feel having made these changes, what is different, was it easy to make the changes? Also monitor how long it took the changes to become new and positive habits.

What's next?

Here is another selection of changes that you might want to try. Aim to incorporate at least four of these over the coming month.

- When choosing your daily fruit, aim to eat as many different colours as possible. Different colours mean different nutrients and the wider a variety of nutrients you nourish your body with, the better.
- The same goes for vegetables. Different colours lead to a more nutritious day.

- If you want to lose weight, cut back your portions by one-quarter. You are unlikely to notice a slightly smaller meal but multiply the effect over many meals and you will see changes in your body.
- Eat slowly. It takes around 20-minutes for your stomach to tell your brain that you are full so by eating slowly you will know to stop when you are full. Eat too quickly and by the time your brain gets the message that you are full, you have overdone it by a long way.
- Have at least one alcohol free day each week.
- Sample a new food product at least once each week. It could be a new vegetable or fruit, a different dressing or sauce, a variation of meat or fish or a different way of preparing a dish. Never stop experimenting.

What do we do with all this information?

You have now gathered a lot of information on different types of food and how they affect you, and on a number of eating strategies and which ones work best for you. There are now three important things to do.

1 Make sure you keep up to date with your food diary, mentally and physically. It is the only guaranteed method of finding out what is really going on and what you want to do about it.

2 Decide your master strategy for healthy eating. Food is for fuel and food can be fun. There is little point becoming obsessive and over-analysing everything you eat, so now that you have gathered the facts about what works for you, make a decision on how much of the time you are going to eat according to your optimum diet plan, and how much of the time you are going to relax about food and drink. This is key to your personal plan for success. Many people operate an 80:20 rule. They eat the best they can for 80 per cent of the time and they relax about food for 20 per cent of the time and, because they have done their research, this gets them the results they want. You might aim for 70:30 or 85:15 depending on what stage of your programme you are at, but whatever balance you choose, pick the correct balance for your current objectives and ensure your chosen balance is sustainable for each period, and in keeping with your short-, medium- and long-term goals.

3 Create your personal daily food checklist to keep you on track at a glance. The checklist contains everything that you know makes for a great day's eating, full of whole-foods, good energy and room for a little flexibility. Daily checklists can then be completed and reviewed as days go by to guarantee you stay on track.

Your weekly food checklist

To compile your weekly food checklist, take all the elements of your food diary that you want to remain in your weekly schedule and list them on a separate piece of paper. Create a column for each day next to each food and drink item and simply keep a record when you have consumed each item for the day. Here is an example.

Item	Day 1	2	3	4	5	6	7
Porridge							
Fruit on porridge							
Fruit during day x 5							
Handful of nuts							
Sandwich lunch							
Salad lunch							
Sushi lunch							
Chopped vegetables							
Dip for vegetables							
Evening protein							
Evening vegetables							
Evening carbohydrates							
Dessert / Chocolate							

Your weekly drinks checklist

Item	Day 1	2	3	4	5	6	7
Water							
Coffee							
Tea							
Mint tea							
Fizzy drinks							
Wine							
Beer							
Spirits							

Checklist notes

- Where fruit features on the checklist, specify the type of fruit in order that you can ensure variety.
- If bread features on the checklist, specify which type of bread.
- When you have more than one option for a particular meal – breakfast, lunch or dinner – list them all for the week and tick which one you went for on each day.
- Assume that all meals are consumed in the correct quantities for your aims – quantities that have been established by your diary. If you eat more than this quantity at any meal, add a '+' sign by the tick in that box.
- Drinks throughout the day can be noted with a tick for each 'portion' or glass or mug. A portion should contain roughly 250 ml. Water will feature heavily on your checklist every day.
- Just because you have wine on your checklist does not mean you have some every day. Decide as part of your master plan how often you want to drink wine during the week and then complete the checklist with the number of glasses on the allotted days. The same is true for fizzy drinks, beer and spirits.

Now use your food diary and your knowledge of what works for you so far to create your own food and drinks checklists.

My weekly food checklist

Item	Day 1	2	3	4	5	6	7

My Weekly Drinks Checklist

Item	Day 1	2	3	4	5	6	7
Water							

When should I use my food diary?

If you are looking to make changes in your fitness and your body shape, you need to monitor what is happening with your food intake. Your diary will show you how your diet affects your performance, energy levels and appearance. Analysing specific meals at specific times enables you to try new approaches. Your diary should be used for experimentation and monitoring the results.

When should I use my food checklist?

Once you are happy with the food choices and schedule that brings you the results you want, transfer your daily requirements to the checklist and use it to ensure you stick to what you know works for you.

Keep using your checklist for as long as you experience the results that you want. If you feel you want to make further changes at any stage, return to your food diary to establish what changes will be beneficial. Once you have discovered your new approach, you can update your checklist.

There will come a time in the future when you are so well practised at monitoring what works for you and making sure it happens that you will no longer need to write everything down. This point marks a new beginning in your attitude to food and your ability to make it work for you. Until you reach this point, continue to use the diary and checklist as guidelines and do not be afraid to return to them at any time in the future.

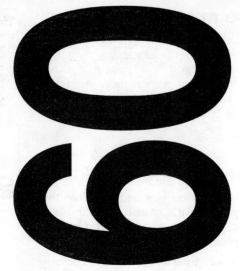

real life fitness

In this chapter you will learn:
- tips to help you stay focused
- techniques to keep you on track
- suggestions on how to maintain fitness as part of your life.

We have explored the notion of not having time for exercise and how to think differently about your fitness, to make it a higher priority and find time to fit it into your timetable. We have also talked a lot about options, being flexible and making sure that when you look at your schedule and see you have got a really busy week coming up, you can still clearly see where you can fit in your activity and healthy eating plans, even if it is not your complete or ideal fitness routine.

Ensuring that you take active steps towards your goals at all times will keep you on track physically and will also reassure you mentally that you are never slipping backwards. A week without exercise or even a few days of food choices that do not work so well for you can play havoc with your mind and make getting started again more difficult than it needs to be. If you have some options of exercises that you can fit into any schedule, you will always feel one step ahead of the game, and as you put together your exercise programmes, you will come up with your own ideas of where you can fit extra activity into your schedule. There are also plenty of ways to sneak exercise into your weekly routine and to experiment with different tricks to keep you on track.

The same is true of your food routine. There may be weeks where it is just not possible to keep to your plan for optimum nutrition but that does not mean you throw caution to the wind. Use your new-found knowledge, experience and skills to work through tricky times and keep yourself headed in the right direction.

Here are some more tips to keep you ahead of the game. You can add your own personal tips to the list as you create them as part of your routine. Then use this section as quick reminders of what you should be doing, and when.

Tips for every day

- Pay attention to how you sit and stand. Just a few days of poor posture and slouching could make you look like you have piled on the pounds, so stand up straight to make your limbs look lithe and toned.
- Plan all exercise sessions well in advance and do not let anything get in the way of them. Decide what you are going to do and when you are going to do it, and then forget about it until the time arrives to get on with it.

- Involve someone else in your exercise plans. Tell people exactly what you are going to do and how you are going to achieve your goals. The more people you tell, the more likely you are to stick to your promises as you will not want to let yourself down by failing to live up to your talk.
- Think carefully about what you are trying to achieve and spend time visualizing how great you will feel when you have achieved it. Plan activities and workouts that will lead you to your results so you know exactly what days and what times you will be exercising. If you plan these times carefully and keep your end goals in mind, you will not talk yourself out of them.
- Find a reliable friend with common goals to exercise with you. By agreeing times and dates to work out you are more likely to see quick results than if you exercise alone.
- Collect photos of yourself – your favourite pictures of yourself as you want to be, and your least favourite pictures of yourself at your worst. Keep them handy with the most favourite on top of the least favourite. Every time you feel tempted to indulge in a food vice, or are struggling to find the motivation to exercise, look at your favourite photos and know that each positive thing you do is a step on the way to getting back to the way you were in the picture.
- Visualize success in the gym and all that goes with it. Think about working out as a key element in creating a new you – a stronger, fitter, healthier, happier you, oozing with self-confidence and sex appeal. The sky's the limit when it comes to imagining the ways in which improving your fitness could improve your life, so think of as many as possible and use them as your motivation to get each workout started.

Kick-starting your progress

- Experiment with new exercises and activities to keep your body and brain stimulated and avoid reaching a training plateau. For one week at the gym, do not allow yourself to use the machines that you normally use. Using different machines will provide a new challenge and you will feel bits working that you never knew you had.
- For one week replace all alcoholic drinks with glasses of sparkling water. Make it as nice a drink as your regular tipple – prepare it as lovingly as you would a gin and tonic with ice

and lemon or lime and really enjoy it. A week of no alcohol will give you a guaranteed reduction in your calorie intake.

- Addicted to coffee shops? See if you can steer clear of them for a week. Go back to basics with a simple cup of tea or coffee and avoid the volume of milk that coffee shops provide and you will also resist the temptations of all the extras that go with it. You will feel lighter and less sluggish and you will save yourself a small fortune in the process.
- Vary your workouts. If you do the same thing every time you go to the gym you will soon reach a plateau in your training and you will get bored. Your body adapts to the workload and soon stops developing so you must always have something in your workout armoury that will keep your body stimulated and continue the great results that you are looking for. Progress leads to more motivation and if you can do your programme easily you are not the master of the gym, you are someone who needs a new workout.
- Have a selection of workouts. You might have an hour or you might only have 20 minutes to spare so you need a workout to suit all occasions. Plan different routines and then keep them in your workout bag so they are always handy.
- Have some back-up plans. If you do feel like a night out, you will need to have a morning-after-the-night-before workout lined up. Providing you can see straight and balance OK you will be fine for some gentle cardiovascular exercise. Go easy on the weights until you feel steady on your feet. A light workout will do you a lot more good that lounging around in bed all day moaning 'never again'. You will feel better generally and doubly virtuous for the fact that you kept your exercise routine going in the face of adversity.

First thing in the morning – tips to get you going each day

- Before you get up in the morning practise tightening your pelvic floor and contracting your tummy muscles while you lie in bed. Hold all the muscles tight for three deep breaths and then relax. Do this ten times each morning and you will be toning up your tummy without even having to stand up.
- While lying in bed, take three deep breaths to get some oxygen into your lungs then tighten your abdominal muscles

and do two sets of 10 gentle crunches before you get out of bed.

- As you get up, sit on the edge of the bed and put a pillow between your knees. Stretch your arms up above you while squeezing your thighs together 15 times to tone your legs.
- When you are out of the bed, take time to make it properly. This is activity that will burn a few extra calories.
- When you are brushing your teeth, make good use of the time by doing some shallow lunges as you brush.

Exercise on the go

- If you travel to work by tube, walk up the escalators two steps at a time. By taking larger strides you will involve your bottom more in your stair climbing and give your legs and lungs more of a workout. If you do not use the escalators you can try this at home in the evening by climbing your stairs 10 times.
- Hold your tummy in and squeeze your bottom, wherever you are.
- If you are waiting for a bus or a train, isolate different muscles around your body and contract and relax them in turn.
- Make every journey a mini-fitness fix. Pick up your pace walking to the station, to the sandwich shop, or even to the wine bar. You will know you have done it right if you are slightly out of breath and can feel your heart racing by the time you get to your destination. Remember this is not about running, just about saying goodbye to the casual stroll and making the most of being on the move.
- If you are in the car, always practise good posture by tightening your tummy muscles and keeping your shoulders relaxed.
- If you spend the day in an office, take regular screen breaks and move around, even if you do not need to go anywhere. Extra journeys mean extra calories burnt which all add up over the course of a day.

Staying on track during the colder months

- Do not hide away under big clothes even when it gets chilly. If you continue to wear fitted outfits then you are more likely to pay attention to your body shape during the winter rather than covering up and hoping for the best when you reveal yourself in the spring. Wear short sleeves at home in the evening to remind you to do a few bench dips off the edge of the sofa while you watch the TV. Two sets of 20 each night is easy and will make a massive difference over a few weeks.

- Design a mini-circuit at home. You do not need much space to create a handy indoor exercise programme that can work all parts of the body without leaving the comfort of your own house. Because of the shorter days, you might not feel like a full workout but a mini-circuit performed a few times a week will give you the same positive results.

- See the winter as an opportunity to try something new. Having a summer fitness routine and a winter routine means that your body is doing different things throughout the year and this will encourage your muscle fibres to remain stimulated at all times rather than reaching a plateau in your training development.

- Buy the right kit. It has been said that there is no such thing as bad weather, only the wrong clothes. If you want to keep your exercise routine intact in the winter, make sure you have all the right gear to protect yourself. Nice new kit is always a good motivator to exercise.

- Change your routine. Early mornings might not be so appealing in the winter so swap to afternoon training to catch the daylight.

- Take out a temporary gym membership to see you through the roughest months.

- Use exercise as your own private heating system. If you get your metabolism fired up you will be warm even on the coldest of days.

- If you train outside in the summer, find the closest indoor equivalent to what you do. So if you run, cycle or row outside in the summer, swap this for treadmill running, indoor cycling and rowing on the machine for the winter.

Holiday fitness

If you cannot get to the gym, try for a single week to get up 15 minutes earlier and do simple stretches and exercises in your pyjamas. Seven days of a few squats, lunges, crunches, press-ups and stretches will boost your energy, set you up for the day and give almost two-hours of exercise in a week.

Family fitness

Many people find themselves in a situation where it is difficult to incorporate fitness into their lives because of family commitments. The only way to work around this is to get everyone involved. This way everyone can spend some quality time together, have fun and enjoy all the positive benefits of getting their bodies moving.

Exercising with your partner

- If you are both members of the gym, set specific times to go together. If you commit to times, you are more likely to stick to the schedule and encourage each other to get there promptly.
- Structure your workout so that you can motivate each other on specific exercises. Shouting at each other may not be that productive, but gentle encouragement and advice on each other's technique can result in a more effective workout for both of you.
- Push each other but work to your own programme. You are not competing but as long as each of you is clear on the other's targets, you can motivate each other to go beyond what you may have thought possible by yourselves.
- Try some new sports together. There is no end of sporting options out there and there is bound to be something that interests you both. It is much more fun to learn something together and as well as spending more time together, the act of trying something new will enrich your relationship.

Exercising with your children

- You can get your children involved in your exercise from an early stage in their lives. Kids love to run around and you should make sure that you join in with them as much as you can.
- Teach your children to ride a bike so that you can all enjoy the freedom of the road together. Cycling is a great skill for them to learn and it also offers them the opportunity to see new places.
- Children love swimming so take them to the local pool and get them started early. You can begin by playing with them in the water and encourage them to swim some widths and lengths so that you can get a workout too.
- Team sports are great for widening a child's social circle and helping them to understand the roles people play in groups. If your children are interested in sport, activities and keeping fit they will understand why it is an important part of your life and will provide you with the space you need for your fitness routine. Because they are also interested, you will have many options for exercising that you can all do together. Your objectives may be different, but you can all take different forms of exercise as a group.

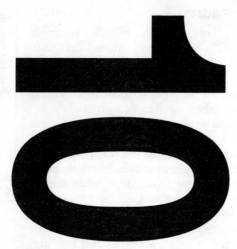

10

fitness forever

In this chapter you will learn:
- that a healthy life is a happy one.

Congratulations on making the effort to read *Teach Yourself Fitness*. You are now armed with all the information you need to get the results you want and to live a long, healthy and happy life. This prospect is reward in itself and we would also encourage you to allow yourself some other rewards along the way to help you with your motivation and keep you on track.

Celebrate success

The satisfaction of achievement is one thing and it can be made sweeter with a little treat now and again. Perhaps a small gift to yourself for completing all your workouts, a massage or treatment to celebrate reaching a particular goal, or some time to yourself to relax or maybe even do nothing. By rewarding yourself you are reinforcing the message that being fit and healthy leads to all sorts of positive feelings and experiences for you. The more often you feel this way, the more likely you are to stick to your plans.

What happens now?

Teach Yourself Fitness contains everything you need for success. We have also included a list of fitness resources and information in the appendix and there are blank copies of questionnaires and paperwork for you to use whenever you need them. You should keep an eye on your progress in the future and when you want to review your situation, return to the book and you will always know where to look for advice, motivation, quick tips and solutions, equipment and other resources. The world of fitness is a large one and there is more information to be found at the research centre at www.the-tonic.com. And if you are really stuck, give one of our experts a call on 020 8995 1302.

Here's to fitness forever ... enjoy!

Getting started

Name:

Date:

Key Fitness Aim

Why do I want to achieve this goal?

By what date will I have achieved this goal?

What will I do to ensure I reach my goal?

When will I start with the New Me?

Setting SMART Goals

What is my fitness priority?

Specific
Write out all details of your fitness priority to make your goal as specific as possible.

Measurable
Describe how you will measure your success with your fitness priority.

Achievable
Is your fitness priority truly achievable by you?

Realistic
Is your chosen fitness priority realistic given your current life circumstances?

Time-framed
Select a time by which your fitness priority will, without any doubt, be reached.

Making your fitness dreams a reality

State your aims in the positive

Where am I now?

What will I see, hear and feel when I reach my goal?

How will I know when I have achieved my goal?

What will reaching this goal get for me?

Is this goal created by me, for me?

What resources will I need to reach my goal?

Is there any cost to anyone else of me achieving my goal?

Is my goal truly exciting, compelling and desirable to me?

Maintaining motivation exercise

Step 1: The truth of the matter

The current situation with my fitness is …

Step 2: Away from motivating triggers

If I continue as I am, the results will be …

If my current patterns of behaviour become more extreme, the most negative consequences could be …

Step 3: Towards motivating triggers

The most important things I want to achieve with my fitness are …

If I make positive changes to my current fitness situation, the benefits will be …

My ideal fitness programme

If I achieved my ideal fitness, what would my life consist of?

What would an average week of fitness look like?

When specifically will I be doing each part of my ideal schedule?

If this is my ideal schedule, with commitments to various activities at set times and days, would it work if I were to put it into action immediately?

Which elements of my ideal fitness programme are possible in reality?

Food diary

Date:

Day:

Time	Food/Meal/ Drink	Hunger rating (0–10)	Moods/Thoughts/ Observations

appendix 6

Exercise diary

Day/Date Time	Exercise/ Activity	Motivation level (0–10)	Enjoyment level (0–10)	Mood Thoughts/ Observations

My personal fitness programme

My Personal Fitness Programme	Exercise	Time/Intensity
Warm-up		
CV training		
Strength training		
Core training		
Flexibility training		

appendix 8

My weekly fitness checklist

Simply insert each activity you intend to do at the head of each column and then tick off the box when the activity is done for that week.

Week					
1					
2					
3					
4					
5					
6					
7					
8					
9					
10					

Your weekly food and drink checklist

Write everything you need to eat and drink in the 'Item' column and simply tick the box when you have consumed each item for the day.

Item	Day 1	Day 2	Day 3	Day 4	Day 5	Day 6	Day 7

appendix 10

taking it further

Fitness resources

Clothing

Sweaty Betty
833 Fulham Road
London
SW6 5HQ
Tel: 0800 169 3889
www.sweatybetty.com
Shop online or at stores
around the UK

Lillywhites
24–36 Lower Regent Street
St James's
London
SW1Y 4QF
Tel: 0870 333 9600

Footwear

Sweatshop
www.sweatshop.co.uk
Shop online or at stores
around the UK

Run and Become
42 Palmer Street
London
SW1H 0PH
Tel: 020 7222 1314
www.runandbecome.com

Equipment and kit

Physical Company
2a Desborough Industrial Park
Desborough Park Road
High Wycombe
Buckinghamshire
HP12 3BG
Tel: 01494 769222
www.physicalcompany.co.uk

Totally Fitness
108 Crawford Street
London
W1H 2JB
Tel: 020 7467 5925
www.totallyfitness.co.uk

Publications

Publications that I have been lucky enough to write for and that always offer sound information and advice on all aspects of fitness include the following. For further published articles visit the press coverage at www.the-tonic.com

Personal Trainer for Women
Vitality House
9 St James Road
Sutton
Surrey
SM1 2BB
Tel: 020 8661 1944
www.personaltrainerforwomen.co.uk

Fitpro Magazine
Fitness Professionals Ltd
Kalbarri House
107–113 London Road
London
E13 0DA
Tel: 08705 133 434
www.fitpro.com

Independent Newspapers
191 Marsh Wall
London
E14 9RS
Tel: 020 7005 2000

Thanks to Independent Newspapers for allowing permission to use source material for the exercise section of this book.

Health & Fitness Magazine
Highbury-WV
53–79 Highgate Road
London
NW5 1TW
Tel: 020 7331 1181
www.hfonline.co.uk

Men's Health
The National Magazine
Company Ltd
National Magazine House
72 Broadwick Street
London
W1F 9EP
Tel: 020 7439 5000
www.menshealth.co.uk

Zest Magazine
The National Magazine Company Ltd
National Magazine House
72 Broadwick Street
London
W1F 9EP
Tel: 020 7439 5000
www.zest.co.uk

Experts

Nutrition and coaching advice

Sarah Tay

Tel: 07976 724 187
www.sarahtay.com

Life Coaching

Upgrade My Life
Tel: 020 8995 9927
www.upgrade-my-life.com

Podiatry, physiotherapy, rehabilitation

Bodyfactor
4 Mercer Street
London
WC2H 9QA
Tel: 020 7420 1440
www.bodyfactor.co.uk

Training organizations

These are training providers that I have studied with and who provide excellent guidance on how to get what you deserve in all aspects of your life.

John Seymour Associates
Park House
10 Park Street
Bristol
BS1 5HX
Tel: 0845 658 0654
www.john-seymour-associates.co.uk

The Performance Partnership
Rosedale House
Rosedale Road
Richmond
Surrey
TW9 2SZ
Tel: 020 8992 9523
www.performancepartnership.com